ASSESSING ANTHRAX DETECTION METHODS

HEARING

BEFORE THE

SUBCOMMITTEE ON NATIONAL SECURITY, EMERGING THREATS, AND INTERNATIONAL RELATIONS

OF THE

COMMITTEE ON GOVERNMENT REFORM

HOUSE OF REPRESENTATIVES

ONE HUNDRED NINTH CONGRESS

FIRST SESSION

APRIL 5, 2005

Serial No. 109–57

Printed for the use of the Committee on Government Reform

Available via the World Wide Web: http://www.gpoaccess.gov/congress/index.html
http://www.house.gov/reform

U.S. GOVERNMENT PRINTING OFFICE

23–142 PDF   WASHINGTON : 2005

COMMITTEE ON GOVERNMENT REFORM

TOM DAVIS, Virginia, *Chairman*

CHRISTOPHER SHAYS, Connecticut
DAN BURTON, Indiana
ILEANA ROS-LEHTINEN, Florida
JOHN M. McHUGH, New York
JOHN L. MICA, Florida
GIL GUTKNECHT, Minnesota
MARK E. SOUDER, Indiana
STEVEN C. LaTOURETTE, Ohio
TODD RUSSELL PLATTS, Pennsylvania
CHRIS CANNON, Utah
JOHN J. DUNCAN, JR., Tennessee
CANDICE S. MILLER, Michigan
MICHAEL R. TURNER, Ohio
DARRELL E. ISSA, California
GINNY BROWN-WAITE, Florida
JON C. PORTER, Nevada
KENNY MARCHANT, Texas
LYNN A. WESTMORELAND, Georgia
PATRICK T. McHENRY, North Carolina
CHARLES W. DENT, Pennsylvania
VIRGINIA FOXX, North Carolina

HENRY A. WAXMAN, California
TOM LANTOS, California
MAJOR R. OWENS, New York
EDOLPHUS TOWNS, New York
PAUL E. KANJORSKI, Pennsylvania
CAROLYN B. MALONEY, New York
ELIJAH E. CUMMINGS, Maryland
DENNIS J. KUCINICH, Ohio
DANNY K. DAVIS, Illinois
WM. LACY CLAY, Missouri
DIANE E. WATSON, California
STEPHEN F. LYNCH, Massachusetts
CHRIS VAN HOLLEN, Maryland
LINDA T. SANCHEZ, California
C.A. DUTCH RUPPERSBERGER, Maryland
BRIAN HIGGINS, New York
ELEANOR HOLMES NORTON, District of
  Columbia

———

BERNARD SANDERS, Vermont
(Independent)

MELISSA WOJCIAK, *Staff Director*
DAVID MARIN, *Deputy Staff Director/Communications Director*
ROB BORDEN, *Parliamentarian*
TERESA AUSTIN, *Chief Clerk*
PHIL BARNETT, *Minority Chief of Staff/Chief Counsel*

SUBCOMMITTEE ON NATIONAL SECURITY, EMERGING THREATS, AND INTERNATIONAL RELATIONS

CHRISTOPHER SHAYS, Connecticut, *Chairman*

KENNY MARCHANT, Texas
DAN BURTON, Indiana
ILEANA ROS-LEHTINEN, Florida
JOHN M. McHUGH, New York
STEVEN C. LaTOURETTE, Ohio
TODD RUSSELL PLATTS, Pennsylvania
JOHN J. DUNCAN, JR., Tennessee
MICHAEL R. TURNER, Ohio
JON C. PORTER, Nevada
CHARLES W. DENT, Pennsylvania

DENNIS J. KUCINICH, Ohio
TOM LANTOS, California
BERNARD SANDERS, Vermont
CAROLYN B. MALONEY, New York
CHRIS VAN HOLLEN, Maryland
LINDA T. SANCHEZ, California
C.A. DUTCH RUPPERSBERGER, Maryland
STEPHEN F. LYNCH, Massachusetts
BRIAN HIGGINS, New York

EX OFFICIO

TOM DAVIS, Virginia

HENRY A. WAXMAN, California

LAWRENCE J. HALLORAN, *Staff Director and Counsel*
KRISTINE McELROY, *Professional Staff Member*
ROBERT A. BRIGGS, *Clerk*
ANDREW SU, *Minority Professional Staff Member*

CONTENTS

	Page
Hearing held on April 5, 2005	1

Statement of:

Burrus, William, president, American Postal Workers Union, AFL–CIO; Linda D. Stetzenbach, director, Microbiology Division, Harry Reid Center for Environmental Studies, University of Nevada, Las Vegas; James H. Schwartz, chief, Arlington County Fire Department; Michael P. Neuhard, chief, Fairfax County Fire and Rescue Department; Philip Schaenman, president, Tridata Division of System Planning Corp.; and John Jester, Director, Pentagon Force Protection Agency, Department of Defense ... 109

    Burrus, William ... 109
    Jester, John ... 164
    Neuhard, Michael P. ... 148
    Schaenman, Philip ... 155
    Schwartz, James H. ... 140
    Stetzenbach, Linda D. ... 117

Rhodes, Keith, Chief Technologist, Government Accountability Office, accompanied by Sushil Sharma, Associate Director for Science, Centers for Disease Control and Prevention; Dr. Tanja Popovic, Associate Director for Science, Centers for Disease and Prevention, accompanied by Maxim Kiefer, Assistant Director for Emergency Preparedness and Response, National Institute for Occupational Safety and Health, Centers for Disease Control and Prevention; Dr. Klaus Schafer, Deputy Assistant to the Secretary of Defense for Chemical and Biological Defense, Department of Defense; Dana Tulis, Deputy Director for the Office of Emergency Management, Environmental Protection Agency, accompanied by Mark Durno, on-Scene Coordinator [OSC] EPA Region 5, Environmental Protection Agency; Thomas G. Day, vice president of engineering, U.S. Postal Service; and Dr. Katherine Kelley, director, Department of Public Health Laboratory ... 12

    Day, Thomas G. ... 73
    Kelley, Dr. Katherine ... 80
    Popovic, Dr. Tanja ... 36
    Rhodes, Keith ... 12
    Schafer, Dr. Klaus ... 55
    Tulis, Dana ... 62

Letters, statements, etc., submitted for the record by:

Burrus, William, president, American Postal Workers Union, AFL–CIO, prepared statement of ... 112
Davis, Hon. Tom, a Representative in Congress from the State of Virginia, prepared statement of ... 8
Day, Thomas G., vice president of engineering, U.S. Postal Service, prepared statement of ... 76
Jester, John, Director, Pentagon Force Protection Agency, Department of Defense, prepared statement of ... 167
Kelley, Dr. Katherine, director, Department of Public Health Laboratory, prepared statement of ... 82
Neuhard, Michael P., chief, Fairfax County Fire and Rescue Department, prepared statement of ... 150
Popovic, Dr. Tanja, Associate Director for Science, Centers for Disease and Prevention, prepared statement of ... 38
Porter, Hon. Jon C., a Representative in Congress from the State of Nevada, prepared statement of ... 61

IV

Letters, statements, etc., submitted for the record by—Continued
    Rhodes, Keith, Chief Technologist, Government Accountability Office, prepared statement of 15
    Schaenman, Philip, president, Tridata Division of System Planning Corp., prepared statement of 157
    Schafer, Dr. Klaus, Deputy Assistant to the Secretary of Defense for Chemical and Biological Defense, Department of Defense, prepared statement of 57
    Schwartz, James H., chief, Arlington County Fire Department, prepared statement of 143
    Shays, Hon. Christopher, a Representative in Congress from the State of Connecticut:
        Letter dated April 1, 2005 187
        Prepared statement of 3
    Stetzenbach, Linda D., director, Microbiology Division, Harry Reid Center for Environmental Studies, University of Nevada, Las Vegas, prepared statement of 120
    Tulis, Dana, Deputy Director for the Office of Emergency Management, Environmental Protection Agency, prepared statement of 65

ASSESSING ANTHRAX DETECTION METHODS

TUESDAY, APRIL 5, 2005

House of Representatives,
Subcommittee on National Security, Emerging
Threats, and International Relations,
Committee on Government Reform,
Washington, DC.

The subcommittee met, pursuant to notice, at 2:07 p.m., in room 2154, Rayburn House Office Building, Hon. Christopher Shays (chairman of the subcommittee) presiding.

Present: Representatives Shays, Porter, Tom Davis (ex officio), and Kucinich.

Also present: Representative Norton.

Staff present: Lawrence Halloran, staff director and counsel; R. Nicholas Palarino, senior policy adviser; Kristine McElroy, professional staff member; Robert A. Briggs, clerk; Andrew Su and Denise Wilson, minority professional staff members; Earley Green, minority chief clerk; and Jean Gosa, minority assistant clerk.

Mr. SHAYS. The Committee on Government Reform, Subcommittee on National Security, Emerging Threats, and International Relations hearing entitled, "Assessing Anthrax Detection Methods," is called to order.

Is this building contaminated? Almost 4 years after mail-borne anthrax attacks killed five Americans, infected 22 others and polluted postal facilities, the answer to that urgent "yes or no" question remains a protracted cacophony of "maybes." Recent detections in local Department of Defense [DOD], mail facilities produced painful reminders of persistent gaps in both the science of biological detection and the art of communicating test results, and risks, to the public.

Today, with those recent events as context and cautionary tale, we assess the extent of progress by Federal agencies toward standardizing and validating sampling, testing and analysis protocols for Bacillus anthracis.

Each incident of suspected or actual biological contamination will be unique. Every situation presents a daunting array of variables and unknowns. But inherent complexity is no excuse to deter needed research or ignore lessons learned in favor of an ad hoc, uncoordinated and scientifically unsound response. All these events pose the same question: Is it anthrax? Is it still there? Only strong science and vigilant integration of that knowledge into a coordinated response will conquer the unknowns and limit the variables that still plague anthrax detections.

(1)

Last year we asked the Government Accountability Office [GAO], to examine anthrax detection strategies used by the U.S. Postal Service [USPS], and other Federal agencies. In a report released today, GAO finds that despite some scattered efforts, the multi-step anthrax detection and confirmation process still has not been validated; that is, scientifically tested to measure its sensitivity, reliability and limitations.

As a result, those responsible for assessing or mitigating anthrax contamination have scant information on which to base selection of sample techniques, specimen storage modes or testing methodologies appropriate to the incident at hand. Nor can first responders, potential victims, or the public have the degree of confidence they need in positive or negative results that only slowly emerge from this loosely forged chain of custody.

Different anthrax detection technologies emitting different measures of "positive" and "negative" can trigger different responses by local, county, regional, State and Federal officials. The public often hears confusing and sometimes contradictory assessments of the anthrax threat. Law enforcement and public health officials on the scene don't get timely, actionable information on the level of risk.

In effect, workers and the public are expected to serve as human detectors, as the absence of illness is used to prove the absence of contamination. But anthrax detection and remediation should be an environmental, not just an epidemiological exercise. Proven tenets of environmental science and industrial hygiene can be applied to determine with measurable accuracy when a building is clean.

Without validated detection protocols, we risk terrorizing ourselves with preventable false positives that subject people to needless countermeasures and, perhaps more dangerously, we invite false negatives that breed an equally false sense of security.

GAO recommends that Federal agencies refine their approach to anthrax detection, build on lessons learned and incorporate probability-based sampling techniques into a more coordinated response. Although these recommendations are directed primarily to the Department of Homeland Security [DHS], it is still not clear who is in charge of this process as evidenced by our crowded witness panels this afternoon.

But the Department of Health and Human Services, specifically the Centers for Disease Control and Prevention, and the Environmental Protection Agency are designated as lead agencies for anthrax detection and remediation. Their testimony today and that of all our witnesses will help us understand how this vital public safety and public health process can be improved. DHS, fully engaged today in the TOPOFF III National Counterterrorism Exercise, will testify at a subsequent hearing.

[The prepared statement of Hon. Christopher Shays follows:]

ONE HUNDRED NINTH CONGRESS

Congress of the United States

House of Representatives

COMMITTEE ON GOVERNMENT REFORM

2157 RAYBURN HOUSE OFFICE BUILDING

WASHINGTON, DC 20515–6143

MAJORITY   (202) 225–5074
FACSIMILE   (202) 225–3974
MINORITY   (202) 225–5051
TTY   (202) 225–6852

http://reform.house.gov

SUBCOMMITTEE ON NATIONAL SECURITY, EMERGING THREATS,
AND INTERNATIONAL RELATIONS
Christopher Shays, Connecticut
Chairman
Room B-372 Rayburn Building
Washington, D.C. 20515
Tel: 202 225-2548
Fax: 202 225-2382

Statement of Rep. Christopher Shays
April 5, 2005

Is this building contaminated? Almost four years after mail-borne anthrax attacks killed five Americans, infected twenty-two others and polluted postal facilities, the answer to that urgent "yes or no" question remains a protracted cacophony of "maybes." Recent detections in local Department of Defense (DOD) mail facilities produced painful reminders of persistent gaps in both the science of biological agent detection and the art of communicating test results, and risks, to the public.

Today, with those recent events as context and cautionary tale, we assess the extent of progress by federal agencies toward standardized and validated sampling, testing and analysis protocols for *Bacillus anthracis*.

Each incident of suspected or actual biological contamination will be unique. Every situation presents a daunting array of variables and unknowns. But inherent complexity is no excuse to defer needed research or ignore lessons learned in favor of an *ad hoc*, uncoordinated and scientifically unsound response. All these events pose the same questions: Is it anthrax? Is it still there? Only strong science and vigilant integration of that knowledge into a coordinated response will conquer the unknowns and limit the variables that still plague anthrax detections.

Page 1 of 3

Last year we asked the Government Accountability Office (GAO) to examine anthrax detection strategies developed by the U.S. Postal Service (USPS) and other federal agencies. In a report released today GAO finds that despite some scattered efforts, the multi-step anthrax detection and confirmation process still has not been validated, that is, scientifically tested to measure its sensitivity, reliability and limitations.

As a result, those responsible for assessing or mitigating anthrax contamination have scant information on which to base selection of sampling techniques, specimen storage modes or testing methodologies appropriate to the incident at hand. Nor can first responders, potential victims or the public have the degree of confidence they need in positive or negative results that only slowly emerge from this loosely forged chain of custody.

Different anthrax detection technologies emitting different measures of "positive" and "negative" can trigger different responses by local, county, regional, state and federal officials. The public often hears confusing, sometimes contradictory, assessments of the anthrax threat. Law enforcement and public health officials on the scene don't get timely, actionable information on the level of risk.

In effect, workers and the public are expected to serve as human detectors, as the absence of illness is used to prove the absence of contamination. But anthrax detection and remediation should be an environmental, not just an epidemiological, exercise. Proven tenets of environmental science and industrial hygiene can be applied to determine with measurable accuracy when a building is "clean."

Without validated detection protocols, we risk terrorizing ourselves with preventable false positives that subject people to needless countermeasures. And, perhaps more dangerously, we invite false negatives that breed an equally false sense of security.

GAO recommends federal agencies refine their approach to anthrax detection, build on lessons learned and incorporate probability-based sampling techniques into a more coordinated response. Although these recommendations are directed primarily to the Department of Homeland

Security (DHS), it is still not clear who is in charge of this process. As evidenced by our crowded witness panels this afternoon, many have a stake in solving the anthrax puzzle.

But the Department of Health and Human Services, specifically the Centers for Disease Control and Prevention, and the Environmental Protection Agency are designated as lead agencies for anthrax detection and remediation. Their testimony today, and that of all our witnesses, will help us understand how this vital public safety and public health process can be improved. DHS, fully engaged today in the TOPOFF III national counterterrorism exercise, will testify at a subsequent hearing.

Mr. SHAYS. At this time, with the lady's permission, I will go to the chairman.

Ms. NORTON. Certainly, sir.

Mr. SHAYS. Thank you.

Chairman TOM DAVIS. Mr. Shays, thank you very much.

I still remember the call I got from Fairfax Inova Hospital in November 2001 telling me that a postal worker from northern Virginia had the symptoms of anthrax. This individual, Leroy Richmond, would ultimately survive inhalation anthrax, but we all remember the five individuals who did not.

Three and a half years have passed since the anthrax attacks on Capitol Hill and millions of dollars have been spent to improve our ability to detect and respond to future anthrax attacks. Yet as both the GAO report released today, and last month's anthrax incident demonstrate, we are still unable to perform those core responsibilities as we should.

In fact, one of my greatest concerns since the United States refocused on homeland security in 2001 has been that we would throw money at innumerable problems to little or no benefit—much sound and fury, signifying nothing. Things are not quite that extreme, but we still struggle to accomplish fundamental tasks, and we must therefore continue to provide close oversight of Federal efforts to better protect our citizens.

As we continue to see, there is little room for error in responding to a real or perceived biological attack. If the situation is not effectively managed, public confidence quickly erodes.

In reviewing the testimony today, it is clear that our ability to detect the presence of anthrax leaves much to be desired. Our response capabilities hinge on our ability to determine whether or not anthrax is present. Proper scientific rigor must be applied to this issue so that all facets of anthrax sampling, strategy development, collection, transportation, extraction and analysis, ensure the highest probability of success.

Last month's anthrax incidents at the Pentagon and Bailey's Crossroads provide an excellent opportunity to assess our ability to respond to a biological attack. While I am pleased the Federal, State and local entities involved conducted, or are conducting afteraction reports, questions have also arisen. Specifically, I am curious why the Department of Defense has developed both detection and response protocols that differ from civilian agencies. I am also curious why DOD did not coordinate medical decisions with the appropriate State and local public health officials.

At first glance it seems that a unified approach across all Federal agencies would be optimal. Is there an operational reason for DOD to be different? If so, what efforts have been made to facilitate interaction with civilian Federal agencies, States and localities?

From my review of last month's events, it seems that even DOD's use of different terminology created much unnecessary confusion, especially when conference calls were the primary means of interagency communication. If our communication methods result in a telephonic Tower of Babel, we are not doing our jobs.

I appreciate the work already commissioned by Virginia, Maryland and the District of Columbia to examine last month's events from the State and local perspective. I eagerly await the Federal component. This cannot be another scenario where lots of people agree that we need to sit down and talk about X and Y. I want to see actions and want to see results.

In closing, I want to thank Chairman Shays for this timely hearing and I look forward to the testimony of our witnesses.

[The prepared statement of Hon. Tom Davis follows:]

Statement of Chairman Tom Davis
Subcommittee on National Security, Emerging Threats, and
International Relations
Assessing Anthrax Detection Methods
April 5, 2005

I still remember the call I got from Fairfax Inova Hospital in October 2001

telling me a postal worker from Northern Virginia had presented with

symptoms of anthrax. This individual, Leroy Richmond, would ultimately

survive inhalation anthrax, but we all remember the five individuals who did

not.

Three and a half years have passed since the anthrax attacks on Capitol Hill,

and millions of dollars have been spent to improve our ability to detect and

respond to future anthrax attacks. Yet, as both the GAO report released

today and last month's anthrax "incident" demonstrate, we are still unable to

perform these core responsibilities as we should.

In fact, one of my greatest concerns since the United States refocused on

homeland security in 2001 has been that we would throw money at

innumerable problems to little or no benefit -- Much sound and fury,

signifying nothing. Things are not quite that extreme, but we still struggle to

accomplish fundamental tasks, and we must therefore continue to provide

close oversight of federal efforts to better protect our citizens.

As we continue to see, there is little room for error in responding to a real or perceived biological attack. If the situation is not effectively managed, public confidence quickly erodes.

In reviewing the testimony today, it is clear our ability to detect the presence of anthrax leaves much to be desired. Our response capabilities hinge on our ability to determine whether or not anthrax is present. Proper scientific rigor must be applied to this issue so that all facets of anthrax sampling – strategy development, collection, transportation, extraction and analysis – ensure the highest probability of success.

Last month's anthrax incidents at the Pentagon and Bailey's Crossroads provided an excellent opportunity to assess our ability to respond to a biological attack. While I am pleased the federal, state, and local entities involved have conducted or are conducting after action reports, questions have already arisen. Specifically, I am curious why the Department of Defense has developed both detection and response protocols that differ from civilian agencies. I am also curious why DOD did not coordinate medical decisions with the appropriate state and local public health officials.

At first glance, it seems that a unified approach across all federal agencies would be optimal. Is there an operational reason for DOD to be different? If so, what efforts have been made to facilitate interaction with civilian federal agencies, states, and localities?

From my review of last month's events, it seems that even DOD's use of different *terminology* created much unnecessary confusion, especially when conference calls were the primary means of interagency communication. If our communication methods result in a telephonic Tower of Babel, we are not doing our jobs.

I appreciate the work already commissioned by Virginia, Maryland, and D.C. to examine last month's events from the state and local perspective. I eagerly await the federal component. This cannot be another scenario were lots of people agree that we "need to sit down and talk about x or y..." I want to see action and results.

In closing, I would like to thank Chairman Shays for this timely hearing, and I look forward to the testimony of our witnesses.

Mr. SHAYS. I thank the chairman. At this time the Chair would also like to recognize another member from the area of D.C., obviously in D.C., who also has vital concerns about this issue.

Ms. Norton.

Ms. NORTON. Well, first, Mr. Chairman, let me thank you for your permission to sit in on this hearing. I am on the full committee, not on your subcommittee, and I appreciate your understanding the special interest that I have in this issue in particular.

I am not surprised, Mr. Chairman, for your foresight, because foresight is what it is, for calling these hearings, and members in this region will think that this hearing is in response to the frightening false alarms that recently occurred here, but this hearing and the GAO report where they were already when that took place makes the hearing especially timely.

Mr. Chairman, I was so concerned, even before we knew that these were false alarms at the Pentagon facilities, that I immediately wrote to Chairman Davis to ask for a hearing, if only to settle the region down. About the last thing this region needs to go through is another sense that we have not gotten control of contamination of the mail, not after we have lost two good men, three others are seriously injured. False alarm or real alarm, the effect on particularly postal employees is virtually the same, and here of course including having to take Cipro.

Mr. Chairman, when I looked at the GAO report, I was absolutely stunned. I could only think what year is this, are we back in 2001, because if you look at that report I think it is fair to say that nothing got fixed. It looks as if everything went wrong—detection, testing, coordination, communication. The only thing that ultimately went right is somebody understood that you ought to at some point tell employees and begin taking steps. Of course, those steps turned out to be unnecessary and we are 4 years after September 11th.

Mr. Chairman, I was particularly concerned that the Pentagon had done its own testing in a non-CDC-certified lab. What in the world is the Pentagon doing farming out this important mission to a lab which hasn't gone through certification by the CDC when there are more than 100 such labs all around the country that have—I couldn't help but think who does the Pentagon think they are? Do they think they are not bound by the rules that came out after the anthrax scare here?

That was extremely disconcerting to me. I cannot know whether or not another lab would have done better. I do know that workers and people who live in this region and in the United States have a right to expect after the anthrax attacks that occurred here and around the country, if I may remind you, have resulted in our taking care of the basics. The basics weren't attended to here and, Mr. Chairman, you were on the case as if clairvoyant with the GAO report and with this hearing, and I can't thank you enough for that.

Mr. SHAYS. I thank the gentlelady and am very grateful that she is here to participate fully in this hearing.

Let me say before recognizing our witnesses and swearing them in, that we have six witnesses in this panel and I think six in the next. So we are going to stick to the 5-minute rule. When the 5 minutes are up, I will ask you to wrap up if you haven't wrapped up, just so we can get to the questions, and we will have a number of questions to ask.

So at this time the Chair would just note for the record that we have Keith Rhodes, Chief Technologist, Center for Technology and Engineering Department, Applied Research and Methods, U.S. Government Accountability Office, accompanied by Dr. Sushil Sharma, just behind him. So, Doctor, if you would stand when we swear and others as well; Dr. Tanja Popovic, Associate Director for Science, Centers for Disease Control and Prevention, Department of Health and Human Services, accompanied by Maxim Kiefer; Dr. Klaus Schafer, Deputy Assistant to the Secretary of Defense for Chemical and Biological Defense; Dana Tulis, Deputy Director for the Office of Emergency Management, Environmental Protection Agency, accompanied by Mark Durno; Thomas G. Day, vice president of engineering, U.S. Postal Service; as well as Dr. Katherine Kelley, director, Association of Public Health Laboratories.

So if you would stand, if everyone else who I called will stand or anyone who might be providing some testimony would stand as well, if there is anyone accompanying you who may participate; if you would all stand and raise your right hands.

[Witnesses sworn.]

Mr. SHAYS. I would note for the record that all our witnesses and those who might testify have responded in the affirmative, and we will start with you, Mr. Rhodes. Thank you very much for being here. I thank all of you for being here and thank you all for your service to our country, whether it's directly in the government or in the case of the Associated Public Health Laboratories for your work as well. Thank you.

STATEMENTS OF KEITH RHODES, CHIEF TECHNOLOGIST, GOVERNMENT ACCOUNTABILITY OFFICE, ACCOMPANIED BY SUSHIL SHARMA, ASSOCIATE DIRECTOR FOR SCIENCE, CENTERS FOR DISEASE CONTROL AND PREVENTION; DR. TANJA POPOVIC, ASSOCIATE DIRECTOR FOR SCIENCE, CENTERS FOR DISEASE AND PREVENTION, ACCOMPANIED BY MAXIM KIEFER, ASSISTANT DIRECTOR FOR EMERGENCY PRE- PAREDNESS AND RESPONSE, NATIONAL INSTITUTE FOR OC- CUPATIONAL SAFETY AND HEALTH, CENTERS FOR DISEASE CONTROL AND PREVENTION; DR. KLAUS SCHAFER, DEPUTY ASSISTANT TO THE SECRETARY OF DEFENSE FOR CHEMI- CAL AND BIOLOGICAL DEFENSE, DEPARTMENT OF DE- FENSE; DANA TULIS, DEPUTY DIRECTOR FOR THE OFFICE OF EMERGENCY MANAGEMENT, ENVIRONMENTAL PROTEC- TION AGENCY, ACCOMPANIED BY MARK DURNO, ON-SCENE COORDINATOR [OSC] EPA REGION 5, ENVIRONMENTAL PRO- TECTION AGENCY; THOMAS G. DAY, VICE PRESIDENT OF EN- GINEERING, U.S. POSTAL SERVICE; AND DR. KATHERINE KELLEY, DIRECTOR, DEPARTMENT OF PUBLIC HEALTH LAB- ORATORY

STATEMENT OF KEITH RHODES

Mr. RHODES. Thank you, Mr. Chairman. Mr. Chairman, members of the subcommittee, thank you for asking us to participate in this hearing by presenting our assessment of the Federal activities conducted to detect anthrax in postal facilities in the fall of 2001.

Mr. Chairman, the bottom line of our findings is the following: Since there were and largely still are no validated methods for sample collection and analysis, agencies cannot know with any level of statistical confidence whether or not a building is contaminated. In short, agencies cannot know when a negative result means negative and when a positive result means positive.

I will now take a moment to discuss two of our major findings about Federal agencies' sampling strategies and lack of validation. Our first finding is that the agencies primarily used a targeted strategy; they collected samples from specific areas considered more likely to be contaminated based on their judgments.

However, such judgments can only be effective when the source of contamination is definitive and the sample collection and analytical methods are validated. In addition, these judgments are based on certain assumptions.

For example, contamination levels at the highest public health concern can usually be detected using a variety of available methods, despite their limitations. However, these assumptions may not always apply. For example, there may be limitations in the available information that restrict an agency's ability to reliably identify target locations. And when all results are negative, additional testing will need to be done, as was the case in Wallingford, CT.

This in turn will result in the loss of critical time needed for public health intervention. A major weakness of targeted sampling approach is that in the case of a negative result, the basic question is this building contaminated will remain unanswered with a given level of confidence.

Without probability sampling, inferences about a facility's status; that is, whether it was contaminated, could not be reliably made based on negative results. Probability sampling would address not only the immediate public health needs but also the wider environmental contamination and cleanup issues.

In the future if the agencies decide to use a targeted sampling strategy, they must recognize that they could lose a number of days if test results are negative. Agencies would then have to collect and analyze additional samples, resulting in a loss of critical time for public health interventions.

As you know, Mr. Chairman, this was the case at the Wallingford postal facility in the fall of 2001. About 3 weeks elapsed between the time the first sampling took place and the results of the fourth testing which revealed positive results. Furthermore, about 5 months elapsed between the time of the first sampling event and the time anthrax was found in the Wallingford facility's high bay area, the rafters above the machine that was contaminated.

Our second finding finds that some collection and analytical methods used by Federal agencies were not validated for anthrax. This means that the agencies had no reliable basis on which to choose one method over another and there can be no statistical confidence in the negative results. Validation as it is generally understood is a formal empirical process involving two steps: One, development of standard protocols and, two, evaluation of those protocols in different labs and on several occasions. Reproducibility of the results by different labs and scientists is an essential component of this evaluation process.

Validating a process is important because operational and health-related decisions are made on the basis of testing results generated by that process. In addition, validation would offer assurance that the results of using a particular method are robust enough to be reproduced regardless of which agency, contractor or laboratory is involved.

Thus, agencies and the public could be reasonably confident that any test results generated by that method were reliable and, in particular, that any negative results would mean that a sample was free from contamination or within the method's limits of detection.

Mr. Chairman, while agencies have taken some actions toward validation, these actions do not address the issue of validating all activities related to sampling. Since the fall of 2001, agencies have begun studies that may contribute to the validation process. Nonetheless, these studies appear to be limited in addressing only some aspect of an individual activity rather than the entire process.

Finally, the agencies have not made appropriate and prioritized investments to develop and validate all activities related to sampling for anthrax and other biothreat agents. Accordingly, we made several recommendations to the Secretary of Homeland Security.

The Secretary should: One, ensure the appropriate validation studies of the overall process of sampling activities, including the methods, are conducted; two, ensure that a definition of validation is developed and agreed upon; three, see that appropriate investments are made in empirical studies to develop probability-based sampling strategies that take into account the complexities of indoor environments; and, four, ensure that appropriate prioritized investments are made for all biothreat agents.

Mr. Chairman, this concludes my statement. I will be happy to answer any questions you or members of the subcommittee may have.

[NOTE.—The GAO report entitled, "Anthrax Detection, Agencies Need to Validate Sampling Activities in Order to Increase Confidence in Negative Results," may be found in subcommittee files.]

[The prepared statement of Mr. Rhodes follows:]

United States Government Accountability Office

GAO

Testimony before the Chairman, Subcommittee on National Security, Emerging Threats, and International Relations, House Committee on Government Reform, House of Representatives

For Release on Delivery
Expected at 2:00 p.m.
Tuesday, April 5, 2005

ANTHRAX DETECTION

Agencies Need to Validate Sampling Activities in Order to Increase Confidence in Negative Results

Statement of Keith A. Rhodes, Chief Technologist, Center for Technology and Engineering, Applied Research and Methods

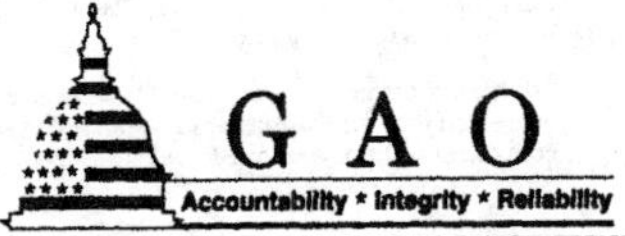

GAO-05-493T

April 5, 2005

Mr. Chairman and Members of the Subcommittee:

We are pleased to participate in this hearing by presenting our assessment of the federal agencies'—U.S. Postal Service (USPS), Centers for Disease Control and Prevention, and Environmental Protection Agency (EPA)—activities conducted to detect anthrax in postal facilities in 2001. My statement is based on our report, entitled *Anthrax Detection: Agencies Need to Validate Sampling Activities in Order to Increase Confidence in Negative Results*, which was issued on March 31, 2005.[1]

As you know, in September and October 2001, contaminated letters laced with Bacillus anthracis, or anthrax spores,[2] were sent through the mail to two senators, Thomas Daschle and Patrick Leahy, and members of the media. The postal facilities in New Jersey and Washington, D.C., that processed the senators' letters became heavily contaminated.[3] Other mail routed through these facilities, as well as additional ones in the postal network, also became contaminated. In addition, numerous federal facilities in the Washington, D.C., area were later found to be contaminated. The letters led to the first cases of anthrax disease related to bioterrorism in the United States. In all, 22 individuals contracted anthrax disease in four states (Connecticut, Florida, New Jersey, and New York) as well as in Washington, D.C. Five of these 22 individuals died.

The threat of bioterrorism has been recognized for a considerable time. Long before the anthrax incidents, several hoax letters indicating the presence of anthrax had been mailed to federal and state agencies, as well as to private sector organizations. In calendar year 2000, the Federal Bureau of Investigation (FBI) responded to about 250 cases potentially involving weapons of mass destruction. Of these, 200 were related to anthrax, although all turned out to be hoaxes. Nevertheless, these events

---

[1] GAO, *Anthrax Detection: Agencies Need to Validate Sampling Activities in Order to Increase Confidence in Negative Results*, GAO-05-251 (Washington, D.C.: March 31, 2005). www.gao.gov.

[2] "Anthrax" in this testimony reflects commonly used terminology. Technically, the term refers only to the disease caused by the microorganism *Bacillus anthracis*, not the bacterium itself or its spores.

[3] Anthrax contamination had been found earlier in several Florida postal facilities that processed mail for the American Media Incorporated building there. However, no letter containing anthrax was ever found.

raised the possibility that facilities could become contaminated and would therefore have to be evaluated for environmental contamination. However, federal agencies have not been fully prepared to deal with environmental contamination, that is, anthrax released through the mail, including the potential for multiple dispersals in indoor environments.[4]

Before I discuss our assessment, let me first present some background. (See appendix I for a discussion of our scope and methodology.)

Background

Although anthrax can infect humans, it is most commonly found in plant-eating animals. Human anthrax infections are rare in the United States, and when infection does occur, it usually results from occupational exposure to infected animals or contaminated animal products, such as wool, hides, or hair. Anthrax infection can occur (1) cutaneously, usually from a cut or abrasion on the skin; (2) gastrointestinally, by ingesting undercooked, contaminated meat; and (3) through inhalation, by breathing aerosolized, or airborne, spores into the lungs.

The response to the incident in the American Media Incorporated building in Florida in September 2001 led to the identification of mail as the potential source of contamination; eventually, it led to the sampling of the postal facilities. The agencies began sampling on October 12, 2001, in Florida and stopped on April 21, 2002, when the Wallingford, Connecticut, facility was sampled for the last time. Four contractors conducted USPS sampling.

The mission of USPS is to provide affordable, universal mail service. As of May 28, 2004, more than 800,000 workers processed more than 200 billion pieces of mail a year. The USPS headquarters office is in Washington, D.C. USPS has nine area offices; approximately 350 P&DCs; and about 38,000 post offices, stations, and branches; the P&DCs vary widely in size and capacity. The USPS mail system is involved in collecting, distributing, and delivering letters, flats (that is, catalogs and magazines), and parcels, as well as other items that vary in size and capacity.

---

[4]According to the head of the Postal Inspection Service, more than 7,000 hoaxes, threats, and suspicious letters and packages—an average of almost 600 a day—were reported to his agency in the weeks following the first anthrax incident. As a result, nearly 300 postal facilities had to be evacuated.

The federal agencies involved in the response in the postal facilities had differing responsibilities. The Centers for Disease Control and Prevention (CDC) and state and local health departments primarily provided public health advice and assistance to USPS. CDC has had primary responsibility for national surveillance of specific diseases, including anthrax; it has also conducted epidemiologic investigations to determine, among other things, the source of the disease. The FBI has been responsible for criminal investigations involving interstate commerce and the mail and crimes committed on federal property. The Environmental Protection Agency (EPA) has been the nation's lead agency for responding to a release of hazardous substances into the environment.

On October 8, 2001, the President created the Office of Homeland Security to develop and coordinate a comprehensive national strategy for dealing with domestic terrorist threats or attacks. The office, which had limited involvement in the 2001 response, was superseded by the Homeland Security Act of 2002, which transferred many of its functions to the Department of Homeland Security (DHS); it became operational in 2003. DHS was created by combining many previously separate agencies and is assigned a lead role in coordinating the efforts of federal agencies that respond to acts of terrorism in the United States.

In addition, the Laboratory Response Network (LRN) was developed in 1999 to coordinate clinical diagnostic testing for bioterrorism. The primary purpose on the biological side was to detect the presence of biothreat agents in a number of specimen and sample types. These laboratories function as first responders that can perform standard initial tests to rule out, but not definitively confirm, anthrax.

Now I will discuss our assessment of the following federal agencies' activities: (1) federal agencies' activities to detect anthrax contamination in the postal facilities; (2) the results of the federal agencies' testing in the postal facilities; and (3) whether agencies' activities were validated and, if not, discuss any issues that arose from the lack of validation and any actions they took to address these issues.

Federal Agencies' Activities to Detect Anthrax Contamination in the Postal Facilities

CDC, EPA, and USPS, the federal agencies involved in sampling the postal facilities in 2001 to detect anthrax, undertook several activities: (1) sampling strategy development, followed by (2) sample collection, (3) transportation, (4) extraction, and (5) analysis of the samples (see fig. 1).

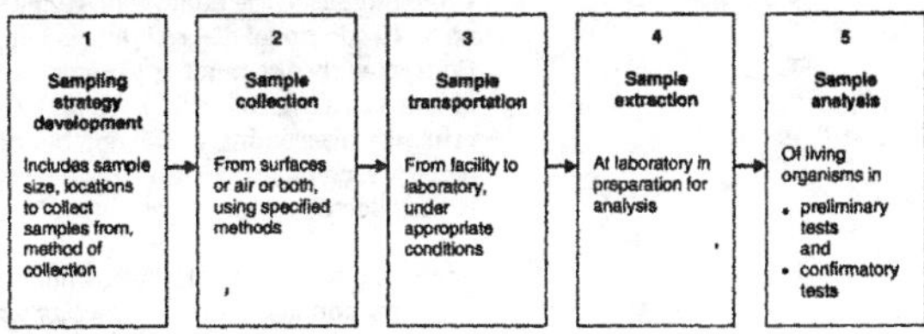

Source: GAO analysis of CDC, EPA, and USPS data.

Neither these activities nor the overall process has been validated for anthrax testing. Consequently, the agencies had only limited information available for reliably choosing one method over another and no information on the limits of detection to use when evaluating negative results. In addition, the sampling strategy used by the agencies could not provide any statistical confidence with regard to the basic question: Is this building contaminated? Therefore, in the future, in the absence of a positive result, a different strategy is needed that will provide statistical confidence, at a defined level, to answer this question.

Activity 1: Sampling Strategy Development

The first activity involved agencies' developing a sampling strategy, which included deciding how many samples to collect, where to collect them from, and what collection methods to use. The agencies primarily used a targeted strategy: They collected samples from specific areas considered more likely to be contaminated, based on judgments. Such judgments can be effective in some situations, for example, in determining (1) the source of contamination in a disease outbreak investigation or (2) whether a facility is contaminated when information on the source of potential contamination is definitive. However, in the case of a negative finding, when the source of potential contamination is not definitive, the basic question—Is this building contaminated?—will remain unanswered.

Agencies Primarily Used a Targeted Strategy

The targeted strategy the agencies used was reflected in their site-specific sampling activities. Sample sizes varied by facility and circumstances, increased over time, and excluded probability sampling. In the beginning, in each USPS facility, 23 samples were to be collected from specific areas relating to mail processing and up to 20 additional "discretionary" samples were to be collected, depending on the type and size of the facility. Later, USPS increased the number of samples required to a minimum of 55, with up to 10 additional discretionary samples for larger facilities. Consequently, the number of samples collected varied by facility, from a low of 4 to a high of 148. CDC's and EPA's site-specific strategies were primarily discretionary. The number of samples CDC collected varied by facility, ranging from a low of 4 to a high of 202. The number of samples EPA collected ranged from a low of 4 to a high of 71.

According to CDC, a targeted sampling strategy may be effective in detecting contamination in a facility when sufficient site-specific information exists to narrow down the locations in which the release and contamination are most likely to have occurred. CDC's assumptions for this strategy are that at the outset, (1) a scenario where all locations have an equal chance of being contaminated is generally the exception rather than the rule; (2) information collected about the event, combined with technical judgment about exposure pathways, can be used to identify locations where contamination is most likely to be found; (3) contamination levels of the highest public health concern can usually be detected using a variety of available methods, despite their limitations; and (4) there is important public health value in quickly identifying contaminated locations. However, these assumptions may not always apply. For example, there may be limitations in the available information that restrict the ability to reliably identify target locations. The method of contamination spread could conceivably be via a mechanism where there is an equal chance of any area being contaminated. Lastly, all results may be negative, which will lead to a requirement for additional testing, as was the case in Wallingford. This, in turn, will result in the loss of the critical time needed for public health intervention.

CDC and USPS officials said that they used a targeted strategy for several reasons, including limitations on how many samples could be collected and analyzed. They also said that in 2001 they lacked the data necessary to develop an initial sampling strategy that incorporated probability sampling. We disagree with this interpretation. Probability sampling is statistically based and does not depend solely on empirical criteria regarding the details of possible contamination.

Incorporating Probability Sampling Would Allow Greater Confidence in Negative Results

We consider probability sampling to be a viable approach that would address not only the immediate public health needs but also the wider public health protection, infrastructure cleanup, and general environmental contamination issues. We recognize that in a major incident, the number of samples that may need to be collected and analyzed may challenge available laboratory resources. Accordingly, there is a need to develop innovative approaches to use sampling methods that can achieve wide-area coverage with a minimal number of individual samples to be analyzed. For example, high-efficiency particulate air (HEPA) vacuum techniques, in combination with other methods, appear to be one such approach that could achieve this. In addition, because of limited laboratory capacity, samples may need to be stored after collection for subsequent analysis, on a prioritized basis.

The situation in 2001 was unique, and the agencies were not fully prepared to deal with environmental contamination. In the future, if the agencies decide to use a targeted rather than a probability sampling strategy, they must recognize that they could lose a number of days if their targeted sampling produces negative test results. In this case, additional samples would need to be collected and analyzed, resulting in critical time, for public health interventions, being lost. This was so at the Wallingford postal facility in the fall of 2001, when about 3 weeks elapsed between the time the first sampling took place and the results of the fourth testing, which revealed positive results. Furthermore, about 5 months elapsed between the time of the first sampling event and the time anthrax was found in the Wallingford facility's high-bay area.

Therefore, in the future, strategies that include probability sampling need to be developed in order to provide statistical confidence in negative results. Further, even if information on all the performance characteristics of methods is not yet available, a probability sampling strategy could be developed from assumptions about the efficiency of some of the methods. And even if precise data are not available, a conservative, approximate number could be used for developing a sampling strategy. This would enable agencies and the public to have greater confidence in negative test results than was associated with the sampling strategy used in 2001.

Activity 2: Collecting Samples

The agencies used a variety of sample collection methods. USPS primarily used the dry swab method. CDC and EPA used premoistened and dry sterile, synthetic (noncotton) swabs, wet synthetic wipes, and HEPA vacuums for sampling. To determine whether anthrax was airborne, CDC performed air sampling in the Brentwood facility 12 days after the contaminated letters were processed. Airborne anthrax spores pose a health risk because they can cause inhalational anthrax, the most serious form of the disease. Agency officials stated that laboratory requirements had influenced the choice of sample collection methods. For example, in the New York area, CDC used only dry swabs, following a requirement by New York public health laboratories.

The majority of the samples were collected by the dry swab method, which experts and others we interviewed considered the least effective. Single methods were involved in 304 sampling events—that is, CDC and USPS collecting dry swab samples (185) and CDC and others collecting premoistened swabs (119).[5] However, for some sampling events, CDC used wet wipes, HEPA vacuum, and air samples at Brentwood and swabs, wet wipes, and HEPA vacuum samples at Wallingford.

USPS officials said that the choice of dry swabs was based on advice from CDC and an APHL working group, which had coordinated with the head of LRN. CDC stated that the reason for the use of swabs was an accommodation USPS had reached with APHL. According to APHL officials, the working group consulted with CDC's NCID in November 2001. APHL said that an NCID official, who was a member of the group, agreed that the dry synthetic swab method could be used but that premoistened swabs would pick up more spores.

During our fieldwork, we tried to determine what specific advice CDC gave the Association of Public Health Laboratories (APHL) on using dry swabs. In responding to our inquiry, CDC did not specifically deny APHL's statement that an official from CDC's National Center for Infectious Diseases (NCID) told APHL that dry swabs could be used. However, an official from CDC's National Institute for Occupational Safety and Health

---

[5] We use "sampling event" to refer to initial sample collection by a specific agency on a specific day and at a specific time in a specific facility. Multiple agencies collected samples on the same day in some of the same facilities; therefore, each agency's sample collection is considered a separate sampling event. As a result, there were more sampling events than the total number of facilities sampled.

(NIOSH), which was not a member of the working group, said that CDC has always recommended using premoistened swabs. Nevertheless, according to APHL, "the NIOSH recommendation was not known by the NCID working group members, nor did they advocate on its behalf."

The decision to use dry rather than premoistened swabs stemmed partly from the concern of some public health officials, including APHL officials we interviewed, that moistened swabs would allow anthrax spores to germinate, growing into vegetative cells instead of remaining as spores. Other public health officials we interviewed said it was highly unlikely that anthrax spores would germinate into vegetative cells in a premoistened swab. APHL officials said that it was feared that such vegetative cells would be destroyed during certain analytic procedures. However, none of the agencies' collection methods were evaluated for anthrax detection in environmental samples. In the absence of empirical research, agencies had no information available for reliably choosing one method over another and no information on the limits of detection to use when evaluating negative results.[6]

Activity 3: Transporting Samples

Agencies transported samples by land or air to laboratories for extraction and analysis (activities 4 and 5). The USPS sample collection plan included shipping instructions that were based on regulations for shipping infectious substances and designed to prevent their inadvertent release. EPA's sample collection plan did not refer to transportation requirements. According to CDC's guidelines, anthrax samples were to be considered infectious substances and packaged according to applicable federal regulations enforced by the Department of Transportation. These regulations were aimed at "ensuring that the public and the workers in the transportation chain are protected from exposure to any agent that might

---

[6]The published literature provided some information on the efficiency of a few sample collection methods. In all the methods studied, swabs were always premoistened before samples were collected. However, according to one study, the most efficient method caused problems when used with certain analytic methods.

be in the package."[7] Among other potential requirements, infectious material must be contained in a securely sealed, pressure resistant, watertight, primary receptacle surrounded by an absorbent and cushioning material. This material must, in turn, be enclosed in a securely sealed, watertight, and durable secondary packaging, which has to be enclosed in an outer packaging constructed of fiberboard or equivalent material, as well as shock absorbent material if more than 50 milliliters are shipped in one package.

However, these regulations did not address one of the most important issues—maintaining the biological integrity of samples while being transported. Failure to do so could result in false negative test results. For example, analysis by culture requires that spores can germinate, divide and multiply, so that tests can determine whether a sample contains anthrax. Temperature and exposure to certain kinds of light, such as ultraviolet light, can be deleterious to some microorganisms. Therefore, it is important that every sample collected retain its original physical form before and during transportation.

We did not attempt to ascertain (1) the specific transit times for delivering all the samples to laboratories, (2) whether sample transportation was delayed, and (3) if it was, how long it was delayed. We also did not attempt to ascertain the environmental conditions the samples were shipped under or when they were received at the laboratories. Finally, we did not attempt to ascertain the degree to which spores could have been exposed to varying environmental conditions from the time of release to the time of sample collection, which could have affected sample integrity. Anthrax spores are robust, compared with other pathogenic microorganisms, but whether transportation affected their viability cannot be known because the conditions of their transportation were not validated. Transport

---

[7]Department of Transportation, 49 *C.F.R.* subchapter C—Hazardous Materials Regulation. The USPS regulations mirror the Department of Transportation regulations. However, to be transported as mail, material must be classified as mailable. By statute, infectious materials, such as anthrax spores, that are "disease germs or scabs, [or] other natural or artificial articles, compositions, or material which may kill or injure another" cannot be mailed. Such materials are termed "nonmailable matter." Knowingly mailing such material is a criminal offense, and doing so with the intent to kill or injure is a felony. When an etiologic material is not "outwardly or of [its] own force dangerous or injurious to life, health, or property," USPS may allow it to be mailed, subject to appropriate rules and regulations governing its preparation and packing. As a result, USPS allows the mailing of small quantities of appropriately packaged infectious material, but only if it is intended for medical or veterinary use, research, or laboratory certification related to public health.

conditions, once validated, would have to be standardized to ensure reproducibility.

Activity 4: Extracting Samples	LRN protocols required that sample material be extracted with specific extraction procedures and fluids (such as sterile saline or water) and that the extracted fluid be subjected to specific analytic methods. For the samples USPS collected under the APHL agreement, the extraction methods included adding a sample processing solution to the conical tubes containing the dry swabs before "plating." This process was adapted from LRN protocols for extracting swabs. However, the private laboratory (not part of LRN) that originally analyzed the samples for USPS did not use an extraction fluid; it inoculated the noncotton, rayon-tipped dry swab directly onto a culture plate.

Several factors could have affected extraction efficiency. For example, according to public health officials and other experts, the degree to which swabs or wipes can retain spores depends on the material they are made of. Cotton is more retentive than some artificial fibers like rayon and may be more difficult for extraction of spores for analysis. Other factors affecting spore extraction are the physical nature of the collection device and surface properties. For example, swabs are easier to manipulate and immerse in extract fluid than more bulky wipes are. CDC has acknowledged that "the recovery efficiency of the analytical methods has not been adequately evaluated."

The reproducibility of the results when an extraction fluid is used can also be an issue. For example, a U. S. Army Medical Research Institute for Infectious Diseases (USAMRIID) official we interviewed told us of an unpublished USAMRIID study conducted to determine the efficiency of extracting anthrax from swabs; the study showed that even if the same procedure was followed, the results were not always the same.[8] Although the importance of reproducibility has been recognized, definitive scientific information regarding extraction efficiency is lacking. In its absence, it is not clear whether sampling results were affected, particularly with respect to samples that may have contained few spores. Without knowing the

---

[8]Using synthetic swabs and a particular type of buffer could lead to 70 to 75 percent extraction. However, repeating the test with the same type of buffer made by different companies yielded different results. The official said that this test showed that there were too many variables. Even when analysts followed the same procedure, the results were not always reproducible, casting doubt on the reliability of the test results.

extraction efficiency, a false negative result may potentially be seen as a true negative.

| Activity 5: Analyzing Samples | Analyzing the samples involved a variety of methods and required two steps—preliminary and confirmatory—to generate a final result. The laboratory analytic methods that were used for detecting anthrax in clinical samples already existed, but they had not been used for environmental samples. As a result, different analytic approaches were taken at the preliminary step, involving adaptations of such protocols. Samples deemed positive at the preliminary step were not always confirmed as positive, as was to be expected. However, this could cause problems for the agencies. In addition, some agencies considered preliminary analyses by field-based instruments unreliable, while others maintained that they were reliable but had been used inappropriately. However, once sample extracts were subjected to the required confirmatory tests, a positive result was indeed a positive. |

In analyzing the postal samples, laboratories used a variety of methods for preliminary and confirmatory testing. Preliminary tests included colony morphology, Gram's stain, hemolysis, and motility tests.[9] Any culture isolates that could not be ruled out in the preliminary step of testing were considered presumptively positive and referred for confirmatory testing. Confirmatory tests included culture analyses (traditional microbiological and biochemical analyses), gamma phage lysis (a test that identifies the susceptibility of the organism to anthrax-specific viruses that create a kill zone in anthrax cultures), and direct fluorescent antibody assay, or antibody analyses employing a two-component test that detects the cell wall and capsule, or outer covering, produced by vegetative cells of anthrax.

Other specialized tests, such as molecular subtyping, were also conducted to determine what strain of anthrax was involved. The test results were reported as positive—anthrax was found—or negative—anthrax was not found. Traditional microbiological analyses require 18 to 24 hours before a result can be generated, depending on the laboratory protocols and

---

[9] When bacteria stained with Gram's stain retained the color of the primary stain (crystal violet), they were considered gram-positive, a characteristic of anthrax. Hemolysis, a procedure involving culturing, identified whether the colonies gave no evidence of red blood cell lysis, a characteristic of anthrax. Motility refers to whether the colonies showed no movement in microscopic observation, another characteristic of anthrax.

procedures. In a few instances, results were also reported as number of colony forming units (CFU) per gram of sample material.

According to CDC guidelines, LRN laboratories were to analyze samples by appropriate LRN protocols. According to CDC, all LRN laboratories were qualified to perform the preliminary tests, and most could perform confirmatory and other specialized tests. While a lower level of LRN laboratory could analyze swab samples for preliminary testing, all other samples—such as bulk, wipes, air samples, or vacuum samples—were to be analyzed at a higher level of LRN laboratory. Samples could also be analyzed at CDC laboratories. Presumptive positives found at a lower level LRN laboratory had to be referred to an appropriately qualified laboratory for confirmatory testing.

The problems agencies encountered in preliminary testing included issues related to training and quality control, as well as problems with using field-based analytic methods with limitations that were not well understood. In preliminary testing, a suspect organism must first be selected; at this point, human error or quality control issues can affect the results. For example, we identified a problem involving culture in the preliminary tests—that is, a reliance on the naked human eye to identify and select the growth of anthrax on the petri dish. Many different types of organisms could be growing that looked like, but were not, anthrax. This is significant because when negative results were obtained during preliminary testing, no further testing was to be done.

The agencies were also faced with problems when deciding how to respond to preliminary positive results that might eventually turn out to be confirmed otherwise. For example, agencies did not have clear criteria for when to close facilities. In addition, although hand-held assays (HHA) were considered preliminary tests, concerns were raised that the negative results might lead to a false sense of security.[10] During the 2001 incidents, USPS kept the Brentwood facility open, following CDC's advice that closing it was not warranted. According to USPS officials, the correctness of this advice appeared to be confirmed by the HHA results obtained on October 18, 2001. When CDC confirmed a case of inhalation anthrax in a Brentwood employee on October 21, 2001, the facility was closed that day. According to USPS, it was not until October 22, 2001, that the laboratory's

---

[10]See GAO, *U.S. Postal Service: Better Guidance Is Needed to Ensure an Appropriate Response to Anthrax Contamination*, GAO-04-239 (Washington D.C.: Sept. 9, 2004).

culture tests of the other samples, collected on October 18, revealed positive results. In a more recent instance, on November 6, 2003, USPS shut down 11 postal facilities in and around Washington, D.C., after a preliminary test—not a confirmed result—from a routine air sample taken on November 5 indicated that a naval mail processing facility might be contaminated with anthrax. USPS tracked the flow of mail through its own facilities and closed 11 postal facilities that delivered mail to the naval facility. The subsequent confirmatory tests were negative, and the facilities were reopened about 3 days later.

All the activities discussed above are interdependent, and many variables for each one can affect the results. Further, problems associated with any one of these activities could affect the validity of the results generated by the overall process. Given that there are so many variables, the use of different sample collection strategies, reflected in site-specific plans, could yield different results. For example, three potential sample collection plans could be used in one facility—plan A, using one collection method (for example, a swab); plan B, using two methods (for example, a swab and wipe); and plan C, using three methods (for example, swab, wipe, and HEPA vacuum). How these collection methods are to be applied—that is, how they are physically used and how much area each sample covers—is a variable. Within each plan, sample transportation protocols could differ, involving variables such as temperature—plans A and B might require transporting at ambient temperature, while plan C might require freezing temperature—the sample collection method's moistness during transport, and the size and construction of the packaging.

In addition, within each plan, laboratory extraction and analysis protocols could differ, involving variables such as (1) different manufacturers' different formulations of extraction fluids, (2) different ways to physically release spores from a particular collection method (such as a swab) into the liquid extract (such as by shaking or vortexing), and (3) a combination of analytic methods, such as culture or polymerase chain reaction (PCR) for deoxyribonucleic acid (DNA) amplification to identify anthrax. Any problems experienced with any of these variables across any of these plans could affect the final result.

The Sampling Results Were Largely Negative

The results of the CDC, EPA, and USPS testing in 286 postal facilities were largely negative. Of 286 facilities, 23 tested positive. For 2 of these 23 facilities, test results were negative at first but positive on a subsequent testing. However, in 1 of these facilities—the Wallingford, Connecticut, facility—it was not until the fourth testing that positive results were obtained.

Testing results differed between the primary facilities and Wallingford. First, in the three primary facilities, results were positive each time a facility was tested, with the important exception of the two quick tests in Brentwood. In Wallingford, considered less likely to be contaminated, results were positive only on the fourth sampling. Second, in the primary facilities, sampling with a single method produced some positive results, regardless of the sample collection method. In Wallingford, neither dry nor premoistened swabs produced any positive results. Third, in the primary facilities, both single and multiple methods produced positive results; in Wallingford, only multiple methods produced positive results.

When comparing the positive results, obtained with dry swabs, across the primary facilities, the proportions differed. For example, in one sampling event in Brentwood, out of 29 samples collected using dry swabs, 14 were positive (48 percent), whereas in Morgan, out of 56, only 7 were positive (13 percent). In addition, for the West Palm Beach, Florida, facility, sampled several times during one sampling event, out of 38 dry swab samples collected, only 1 was positive (about 3 percent). While we did not define this facility as primary, it was suspected of processing a contaminated letter, although none was found. However, the use of both wet and dry swabs produced positive results in this facility.

USPS and CDC sampled facilities that processed mail from the primary facilities to determine whether any other facilities had become contaminated. The majority of test results from these facilities were negative: Of 286 facilities sampled, 23 tested positive, including the 3 primary facilities, and 263 tested negative.

For some of the positive facilities, excluding the primary ones:

- Generally, only 1 or 2 of the total samples collected for each facility were positive, such as several post offices that received mail from Brentwood, including Dulles (11 samples collected, 1 positive), Friendship Station (32, 1 positive), Pentagon Station (17, 2 positive), and Raleigh, North Carolina (42, 1 positive). These facilities were considered cross-contaminated.

- West Palm Beach and Wallingford tested positive only on retesting, whereas initially they had tested negative. The West Palm Beach facility tested positive on the second testing. According to CDC, the sampling strategy used in this facility was found to have limitations and was not used again. However, Wallingford did not test positive until the fourth testing. These results underscore the importance of retesting and cast doubt on the efficiency of the testing.

Of the 263 facilities that tested negative, only 9 were sampled more than once. A facility in West Trenton tested negative, even though an employee had contracted cutaneous anthrax. The facility in West Trenton was tested twice by the FBI and once by CDC, during which a total of 57 samples were collected, with negative results.

Final, or confirmed, results will be negative if contamination is not present in a facility. However, a result can be negative for several other reasons, such as (1) the sampling method was not efficient enough, (2) samples were not collected from places where contamination was present, (3) not enough samples were collected, (4) not enough spores were recovered from the sample material, or (5) analysis of the sample extract was not sensitive enough to detect anthrax spores that were present (that is, the result was a false negative).

Agencies' Activities Were Not Validated

None of the agencies' activities to detect anthrax contamination in the postal facilities were validated. Without validation, the sampling activities could have been based on false assumptions. Using an ineffective method or procedure could result in a finding of no contamination when in fact there is contamination—a false negative. Because the sampling methods are not validated, it is not known to what extent they will underestimate contamination. Thus, in the case of a negative result, agencies would have no sound basis for taking public health measures for the occupants of the contaminated facility.

Validation, as it is generally understood, is a formal, empirical process in which the overall performance characteristics of a given method are determined and certified by a validating authority as (1) meeting the requirements for the intended application and (2) conforming with applicable standards. Because the agencies did not use an empirical process to validate their testing methods, the agencies had limited information available for reliably choosing one method over another and no information on the detection limit to use when evaluating negative results.

Validating the overall process is important because operational and health-related decisions are made on the basis of testing results generated by that process. In addition, validation would offer assurance that the results of using a particular method, which is part of that process, are robust enough to be reproduced, regardless of which agency, contractor, or laboratory is involved. Thus, agencies and the public could be reasonably confident that any test results generated by a process that includes that method would be reliable and, in particular, that any negative results would mean that a sample was free from contamination (within the method's limits of detection).

In preparing for future incidents, the agencies have (1) made some changes based on what has been learned about some of the limitations of their sampling strategies, (2) made some revisions to their guidelines to reflect some of this knowledge and experience or developed new ones, (3) funded some new research, and (4) planned or conducted conferences addressing some of the issues we have identified. In addition, DHS has taken on the role of coordinating agencies' activities and has undertaken several new initiatives related to dealing with anthrax and other biothreat agents.

However, while the actions DHS and other agencies have taken are important, they do not address the issue of validating all activities related to sampling. Since the fall of 2001, studies have been performed, or are under way, that may contribute to the validation of the individual activities. Nonetheless, these studies address only some aspects of an individual activity rather than the overall process. Finally, the agencies have not made appropriate and prioritized investments to develop and validate all activities related to anthrax and other biothreat agents.

Conclusions

The lack of validated methods for assessing contamination in postal facilities impeded the agencies in responding to the incidents. The need that all methods, from sampling to final analysis, be validated, so that their performance characteristics can be clearly understood, is not in doubt. But any combination of methods that makes up the overall process should also be validated because the effect of different permutations of methods may not be predictable. It must be recognized, however, that an inability to validate the entire process reduces, to some degree, the level of confidence in the results. To assess the impact of relying on the validation of individual activities, experiments could be performed with a limited number of processes, combining different methods.

The issues we have raised in this report apply to any anthrax incident, including the March 2005 incident involving DOD facilities in the Washington, D.C. area. In addition, while the 2001 events involved anthrax, many other biothreat agents exist. Differences in their characteristics mean different solutions. Accordingly, efforts to develop sampling strategies and to validate methods should address requirements specific to those biothreat agents as well. However, since addressing other agents would consume resources and time, these efforts should be prioritized in a long-term strategy.

The several agencies that dealt with the anthrax attacks generally worked well together, but we have identified areas that would have benefited from one agency's taking the lead in coordinating the response. Given the mission of DHS and its responsibilities, it appears that DHS is now well positioned to take a lead role in promoting and coordinating the activities of the various agencies that have technical expertise related to environmental testing. In addition, it is important that all participating agencies recognize and support DHS in that role and that they have an effective structure for participating in identifying and addressing the appropriate issues.

Recommendations for Executive Action

Accordingly, in our report, we recommended that to improve the overall process for detecting anthrax and to increase confidence in negative test results generated by that process, the Secretary of Homeland Security develop a coordinated approach. This approach would include working with agencies to ensure that appropriate validation studies of the overall process of sampling activities, including the methods, are conducted. Specifically, the Secretary should (1) take a lead role in promoting and coordinating the activities of the various agencies with technical expertise related to environmental testing; (2) ensure that a definition of validation is developed and agreed on; (3) guarantee that the overall process of sampling activities, including methods, is validated so that performance characteristics, including limitations, are clearly understood and results can be correctly interpreted; (4) see that appropriate investments are made in empirical studies to develop probability-based sampling strategies that take into account the complexities of indoor environments; (5) ensure that appropriate, prioritized investments are made for all biothreat agents; and (6) ensure that agency policies, procedures, and guidelines reflect the results of such efforts.

We obtained written comments on a draft of this report from CDC, DHS, and USPS. We also obtained written comments from APHL on excerpts from the draft that pertained to its role in anthrax testing. Although we requested comments from DOD and EPA, DOD said it had no comments and EPA provided only technical comments.

CDC, DHS, and USPS, as well as APHL, agreed with our conclusion—methods for detecting anthrax contamination in facilities were not validated—and with the thrust of our recommendations—calling for a coordinated, systematic effort to validate the methods to be used for such testing.

In response, DHS stated that while it has the overall responsibility for coordination for future biological attacks, EPA has "the primary responsibility of establishing the strategies, guidelines, and plans for the recovery from a biological attack while HHS has the lead role for any related public health response and guidelines." DHS further stated that EPA "is developing specific standards, protocols, and capabilities to address the risks of contamination following a biological weapons attack and developing strategies, guidelines, and plans for decontamination of persons, equipment, and facilities." DHS pointed out that in the Conference Report on H.R. 4818, the conferees expressed their expectation that EPA will

enter into a comprehensive MOU [memorandum of understanding] with DHS no later than August 1, 2005 that will define the relationship and responsibilities of these entities with regard to the protection and security of our Nation. The Conferees expect the MOU to specifically identify areas of responsibilities and the potential costs (including which entity pays, in whole or part) for fully meeting such responsibilities. EPA shall [is to] submit to the House and Senate Committees on Appropriations a plan no later than September 15, 2005 that details how the agency will meet its responsibilities under the MOU, including a staffing plan and budget.

Finally, DHS stated, "Even though DHS is in charge during a biological attack, EPA is primarily responsible for the coordination of the recovery process. So, DHS will coordinate with EPA to ensure appropriate investments are made to explore improved sampling." With respect to our recommendation that DHS develop probability-based sampling strategies, DHS said that it must first define the necessary requirements for the sampling process and then evaluate targeted and probability-based sampling strategies against those requirements. DHS said that targeted sampling may be beneficial for some applications. We agree with DHS on the need to define the requirements for the sampling process and to evaluate sampling approaches against those requirements. On the basis of the work we have done on this review, we believe that (1) DHS will find that targeted sampling will not always meet all the requirements to answer the question of whether a facility is contaminated and (2) probability-based sampling will be necessary when information on the source and path of potential contamination is not definitive. In our view, probability sampling will be necessary in order for DHS to achieve its goal of having a "scientifically defensible sampling strategy and plan."

Mr. Chariman, this concludes my prepared statement. I will be happy to answer any questions you or Members of the Subcommittee may have.

Contacts and Acknowledgments

If you or your staff have any questions about this report or would like additional information, please contact me at (202) 512-6412, or Sushil Sharma, PhD., DrPH, at (202) 512-3460. We can also be reached by e-mail at rhodesk@gao.gov and sharmas@gao.gov.

Other staff that contributed to this report include Hazel Bailey, Heather Balent, Venkareddy Chennareddy, Crystal Jones, Jack Melling, Penny Pickett, Laurel Rabin, Mark Ramage, and Bernard Ungar.

Appendix I: Scope and Methodology

To respond to your request, we interviewed officials from federal agencies involved in sampling the postal facilities. The federal agencies included the Centers for Disease Control and Prevention (CDC), the Environmental Protection Agency (EPA). We also interviewed U.S. Postal Service (USPS), Association of Public Health Laboratories (APHL), public health and private sector laboratories, and experts on microbial detection in indoor environments.

We reviewed documentation provided or developed by CDC, EPA, and USPS, including sample collection strategies, guidance, environmental collection and analytical methods and protocols. In addition, we reviewed and analyzed test results data, that is, sample collection and analytical data collected by federal agencies, their contractors, and public health laboratories. We did not independently verify these data.

We conducted site visits to some postal facilities affected by anthrax and some public health and private sector laboratories that were involved in analyzing samples. We also reviewed studies on sampling methods for detecting biological substances, including anthrax, on surfaces and in the air. We conducted our review from May 2003 through November 2004 in accordance with generally accepted government auditing standards.

Although our study focused on anthrax testing relating to 2001 anthrax incident, we believe that the issue we identified concerning the need for validated methods and sound sampling strategies would apply to similar incidents in future. This is particularly evident given the consequences arising from the March 2005 incident involving facility closures following preliminary anthrax testing in the Washington, D.C. area.

Mr. SHAYS. I didn't interrupt you because you left your most important part to the end and I couldn't interrupt you.

Mr. RHODES. Thank you very much, Mr. Chairman.

Mr. SHAYS. You are welcome.

Dr. Popovic.

Dr. POPOVIC. Thank you very much.

Dr. SHAYS. Is your mic on, Doctor?

Dr. POPOVIC. It is now.

Mr. SHAYS. Good.

STATEMENT OF DR. TANJA POPOVIC

Dr. POPOVIC. Good afternoon, Chairman Shays and members of the subcommittee. I am Dr. Tanja Popovic, Acting Associate Director for Science for Disease Control and Prevention, and I am accompanied today by Mr. Max Kiefer of CDC's National Institute for Occupational Safety and Health.

On behalf of CDC, I am pleased to describe CDC's views on detection of anthrax, the role of the laboratory response network and our ongoing activities to fully establish the scientific validity of environmental testing methods.

During the 2001 anthrax attacks, CDC teams conducted a number of outbreak investigations in Florida, New York City, New Jersey, Washington, DC, and Connecticut. An environmental sampling was a very important component of these investigations.

CDC used targeted or epidemiologically driven sampling strategies as the most straightforward approach to initial assessment that allowed for rapid determination of contamination and quick public health decisions. Targeted sampling proved to be rapid, efficient and successful and will continue to be our primary strategy in outbreak investigations.

Environmental sampling approaches have substantially expanded since that time, and now they include early warning systems. BioWatch is an environmental air sampling surveillance initiated by the Department of Homeland Security with CDC, Department of Justice, EPA and National Laboratories as key partners. Over 500,000 analyses have already been conducted. Another system is biohazard detection system, the one used by the U.S. Postal Office, postal system. Both of them rely on a phased-in approach, and that is the initial signal for a particular biothreat agent is then followed by confirmatory identification.

CDC has worked very closely with USPS and public health partners on steps needed for that confirmatory identification and on developing effective response protocols. CDC has also taken the lead in working with Department of Homeland Security, Department of Justice and EPA in creating similar guidance for response to BioWatch signals. It is exactly the highly reliable methods of the Laboratory Response Network [LRN], that are used for this step of confirmatory identification.

LRN is a national network of front line and advanced laboratory capacities capable of providing support in bio-threat, chemical or other public health emergencies. During 2001, LRN laboratories have conducted hundreds of confirmatory identifications for anthrax bacteria from all kinds of sources, environmental, human and others. They have also tested more than 120,000 environmental specimens for a total of about 1 million tests. At this time, it is very important for us to continue to grow and enhance this network's capacity to be parallel with its continuously growing responsibilities.

With much of the progress, CDC does agree with the GAO that there is room for further research in the area of validation. The anthracis protocols that we used in 2001 have been validated for identification of the anthracis, and the members of the participating laboratories did take part in the proficiency testing programs.

However, validation methods for collecting Bacillus anthracis from air and surface did not exist at that time and therefore CDC used caution when providing recommendations and guidance for use of these methods to others. We began addressing the issues of validation of these methods immediately after the response ended. And the example of that is a side-by-side study conducted at Brentwood in which we used different sampling materials, which was done almost in the middle of the national crisis.

We do continue to make efforts to validate components of this biothreat agent detection process, but we do believe that the full validation of every possible scenario variation might not only be practical but could not entirely replace the scientific judgment and event-specific evaluations.

In the meantime, CDC microbiologists have really worked hard on evaluating efficiency of different sampling materials and processing methods. We had an interagency agreement with the U.S. Army Dugway Proving Grounds that has led to the development of a chamber in which we can establish and generate known concentrations of anthrax spores, which is critical for any kind of reliable and repetitive validation procedures. Studies are under way that will look at the efficiency of sampling methods for both air and surfaces that will allow for the detection—for lower limits of detection and also, very importantly, talk about intra-laboratory validation.

We also have extensive collaboration with the Sandia National Laboratory on a project funded by DHS, and these are the studies that will talk about the surface sampling and extraction methods as well.

So, in summary, environmental microbiology and sampling issues are indeed important tools for public health decisions, for law enforcement investigations and for evaluation of remediation success. CDC is sponsoring research for a number of validation gaps for Bacillus anthracis, and there are many other agents, and we are looking forward to working with all the agencies, Department of Health and Human Services, Homeland Security and other agencies, so that we can move forward and improve all of our methods.

[The prepared statement of Dr. Popovic follows:]

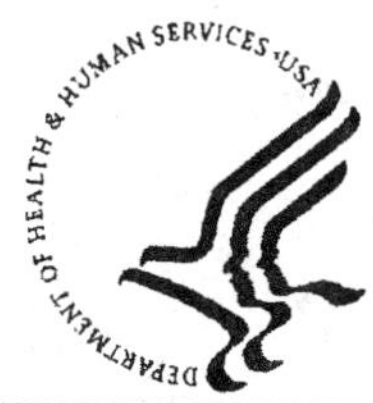

Testimony
Before the Committee on Government Reform
Subcommittee on National Security, Emerging
Threats, and International Relations
United States House of Representatives

Assessing Anthrax Detection Methods

Statement of

Tanja Popovic, M.D., Ph.D.
Acting Associate Director for Science
Centers for Disease Control and Prevention
U.S. Department of Health and Human Services

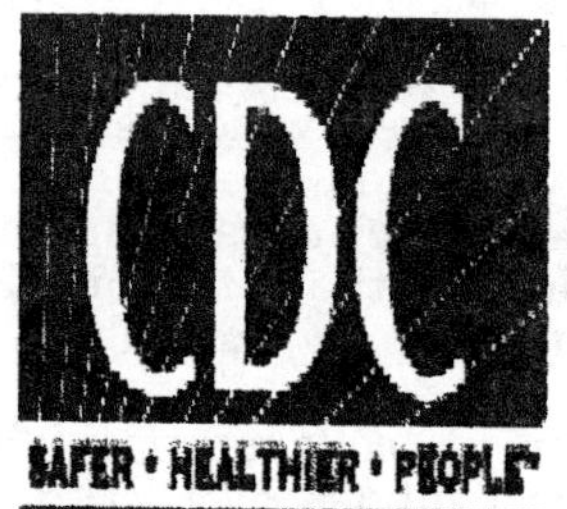

For Release on Delivery
Expected at 2:00PM
Tuesday, April 5, 2005

Good afternoon, Chairman Shays and members of the Subcommittee. I am Dr.
Tanja Popovic, Acting Associate Director for Science with the Centers for
Disease Control and Prevention (CDC). Accompanying me today is Mr. Max
Kiefer, Assistant Director for Emergency Preparedness and Response for CDC's
National Institute for Occupational Safety and Health (NIOSH). On behalf of
CDC, I am pleased to provide this testimony describing our views on validation
issues, our work with the United States Postal Service (USPS) detecting anthrax
contamination during the bio-terrorism attacks of 2001, and ongoing research
and developments to improve environmental testing methods.

CDC is part of the Department of Health and Human Services (HHS). As the
nation's disease prevention and control agency, CDC's responsibility is to
provide national leadership in the public health and medical communities in a
concerted effort to detect, diagnose, respond to, and prevent injury and illnesses,
including those that occur as a result of a deliberate release of biological agents.

During the anthrax attacks of 2001, CDC assumed a wide range of
responsibilities including surveillance to detect new cases of illness;
epidemiologic investigations to assess the risks of infection; collection of
environmental samples to determine the extent of contamination in affected
buildings; analysis of environmental and clinical laboratory specimens; delivery of
stockpiled antibiotics and vaccine; follow-up of persons receiving stockpile

products; and communication with the public and with public health professionals to provide up-to-date guidance and recommendations.

Once the emergency phase was complete, CDC published peer-reviewed reports on each of the outbreak investigations to share findings and improve scientific understanding of bio-terrorism incidents. CDC initiated research to improve our environmental sampling tools and provided technical advice on environmental sampling and related issues to the Environmental Protection Agency (EPA) and others working to remediate and restore anthrax-contaminated buildings.

Since 2001, CDC has collaborated with other agencies on several new efforts. For example, CDC worked with the Departments of Homeland Security and Justice and the Environmental Protection Agency in developing the draft BioWatch Preparedness and Response Guidance, a three part tool that provides guidance for preparedness, response and environmental sampling as it pertains to this environmental surveillance effort initiated by the Department of Homeland Security (DHS). This draft guidance was created in collaboration with, and has been approved by HHS, DHS, Department of Justice (DOJ), and EPA. CDC is working with DHS and national laboratories on issues related to restoration of public transportation systems in the event of a bio-terrorist act. In sum, CDC has worked to improve preparedness and prevention capabilities and has worked with other government agencies to enhance coordination and fill research gaps.

The invitation letter from the Subcommittee asked CDC to address a number of

technical environmental sampling issues.   Our comments on these various

issues are provided below.

Environmental sampling

Environmental testing of potentially contaminated facilities played an important

role in the 2001 CDC response. Subject matter experts at CDC guided efforts to

collect and analyze surface, bulk, and air samples for *Bacillus anthracis*. CDC

consulted with military and other experts and revised guidance for conducting

environmental sampling and lab analysis based on the best available information

and incorporation of ongoing experience. Existing programs, such as the

Laboratory Response Network (LRN), which links state and local public health

laboratories with advanced capacity laboratories, were strengthened in the

enormous effort to enlist resources to identify potential contamination. During the

anthrax attacks, LRN laboratories tested more than 125,000 environmental

specimens alone, which represented over 1 million individual laboratory tests.

Environmental sampling helped identify the likely source of infection and exclude

alternative sources. It improved CDC's understanding of environmental

exposure pathways, including the potential for re-aerosolization of spores and

informed decisionmaking about chemoprophylaxis of exposed individuals,

remediation, and re-occupancy.

The concept of environmental sampling has expanded since 2001 to include the development of early warning systems to provide a signal should a new event occur. These new systems rely on a phased approach. Detection of suspect bio-agents via ongoing sample collection and analysis is the first phase. Biowatch or the USPS "Biohazard Detection System (BDS)" are examples of such systems. Identification is the second phase. It involves confirmation via high-reliability LRN laboratory testing to confirm and identify the presence of a bio-agent. Additional sampling by law enforcement and public health representatives may occur during the investigation/response phase to further guide interventions. These systems work in parallel with the national health monitoring initiative known as "BioSense" which monitors illness trends to provide additional early detection capability to our national public health system.

Validation

The term validation is used by environmental sampling experts to describe quality assurance testing needed to determine the reliability of a given method. It generally involves comparing the performance of a method against either a "reference method" or a known concentration to establish the precision, accuracy, and the upper and lower limits of the method. Environmental testing generally involves at least a sample collection step and a sample analysis step to identify the presence of an agent and, if possible, an estimate of the amount present. No method allows 100% recovery of an agent. Validation is often done in steps and methods that show promise after early testing may receive more testing to address issues such as inter-lab variability.

At the time of the 2001 bio-terrorism events, the LRN sample analysis protocols used to identify *B. anthracis* had been validated, and member labs participated in a proficiency testing program. These LRN protocols were used for analysis of both clinical and environmental samples and had been validated for processing and detecting *B. anthracis* spores. In addition, evidence demonstrated that the spores would most likely not be affected by various shipment methods. In 2001, data were available to suggest that light and temperatures encountered in transport would not have negatively affected anthrax spore viability.

However, validated methods for sample collection of *B. anthracis* via surface or air sampling did not exist at that time. Because of this, CDC used caution when interpreting results from these methods, and CDC included explicit messages about the lack of validation on all sampling guidance used internally and shared with other governmental partners.

While the available sample collection methods lacked validation for *B. anthracis*, established methods had been validated for sampling of other biological agents. Existing methods were extrapolated to the collection of anthrax spores in consultation with subject matter experts.

CDC began planning for quality assurance testing for these methods shortly after the emergency response phase ended. Validation for biological agents is complicated because it involves dealing with living systems. Not all cells will respond or grow given the same nutrients, humidity, and temperature conditions. Reliably creating known concentrations of spores on surfaces and in air for validation studies is a time-consuming technical challenge. In addition, validation for bio-terrorism agents is especially challenging as there are limited facilities to do such studies. As a result of these complexities, it would not have been technically possible for CDC to validate sampling methods during the anthrax attack response in 2001.

CDC partnered with USPS in a research project to utilize existing contaminated surfaces at postal facilities for comparing the collection capabilities of surface sampling methods. These "side-by-side" tests performed in December 2001, sought to overcome the time consuming technical challenges associated with generating known surface contamination levels in a laboratory. The side-by-side tests scientifically compared each of the key methods to other methods and provided an important objective basis for method selection. While this research did not equal "comprehensive" validation, it directly addressed the most important data gaps associated with method selection. Similar testing involving air sampling was performed at the USPS Trenton facility shortly after the public health emergency in February 2002.

Detecting anthrax contamination in Postal facilities

CDC performed outbreak investigations in Florida, New York, New Jersey, Washington, D.C., and Connecticut in response to disease cases resulting from the anthrax attacks. Each investigation involved a multi-disciplinary public health team that included CDC and local and state health department representatives. Teams coordinated closely with USPS and law enforcement representatives. Environmental sampling was integrated into each outbreak investigation. The purpose of these investigations was to identify the source of exposure and to determine if additional public health interventions were needed (e.g. antibiotic prophylaxis, vaccines, facility closures). Outbreak-related sampling was performed in three types of settings: 1) facilities where postal employees at the facility contracted anthrax (e.g. Trenton and Brentwood); 2) facilities that were part of epidemiologic investigations looking for clues on the role that cross-contaminated mail may have played in non-postal employee cases; and 3) facilities where sampling, epidemiologic, or mail flow patterns suggested cross-contamination of mail may have resulted in their contamination (e.g. all 50 post offices upstream/downstream of the Trenton sorting facility). CDC tested 112 facilities and found 12 facilities with positive results. Another seven facilities in Florida were sampled in collaboration with the Environmental Protection Agency (EPA) – all seven involved positive results. Surface testing involved methods such as swabs, wipes, and vacuum sock samples.

Sampling strategies

CDC used targeted (also known as epidemiologically driven) sampling strategies during the outbreak investigations to determine where to collect environmental samples. Incident-specific details (epidemiologic data, interviews with USPS personnel, and understanding of the mail handling process) were used to help identify locations considered most likely to be contaminated so that environmental samples could be collected at these locations. This "worst case" approach used well-accepted empirical approaches to identify plausible contamination pathways. The primary objective in most cases was to maximize the possibility of finding contamination. For example, targeted sampling utilized postal code information printed on the recovered Daschle letter envelope to identify that Brentwood Delivery Bar Code Sorter (DBCS) #17 had processed the letter. Machine #17 was sampled and specific attention was given to locations closest to #17's mail path.

CDC believes that a targeted sampling strategy is the most rapid, efficient, and successful approach when information is available on the path of the terrorism source or vehicle. Targeted strategies not only produced the highest probability of identifying a positive sample during the 2001 response, but also helped to establish locations that posed the greatest risk of exposure.

Targeted sampling must be supplemented with other approaches when there is a lack of incident information to direct samples. Full inspection approaches, where 100 percent of a type of surface is targeted may also be needed. In addition,

CDC believes there is a need to further develop probabilistic sampling approaches (i.e. using random sampling and statistical inferences) to provide additional sampling strategy tools.

Evaluating the meaning of environmental sampling results

Several factors fostered CDC's confidence in interpreting and evaluating environmental sampling results during and after the 2001 events. The methods led rapidly to successful collection of positive anthrax samples during the investigations. Experienced industrial hygienists trained to recognize and evaluate complex hazardous environments were used to perform the sampling. Routine advance communication between the industrial hygienists collecting the samples and the LRN Level B laboratory experts analyzing the samples ensured mutual understanding on sampling methods, sample numbers, shipment, and analysis. In the absence of validated methods specifically for anthrax, these factors and this teamwork model strengthened CDC's confidence in the results obtained from testing.

Furthermore, CDC used care in evaluating the meaning of sample results. CDC understood that results would be "qualitative" (positive/negative) and that there were no available health based criteria for evaluating environmental contamination levels. As a result, no formal criteria were used to further distinguish among positive results. CDC also understood that air sample results collected some time after facility closure might be negative and that surface samples were more reliable indicators of contamination after the fact.

CDC emphasizes that environmental sampling information was not used in isolation but in conjunction with other outbreak investigation information such as epidemiology findings and facility engineering and work practice information. At times, interventions were recommended based on the larger picture despite a lack of positive environmental results. Care was used in interpretation of "negative" test results given the recognition that the lowest limit of detection (i.e. the minimum concentration of anthrax spores that can be detected) for the methods was not available. For example, local illness surveillance activities were continued to provide alternative sources of information.

Based on GAO's recommendation during the May 2003 Congressional hearings, CDC also worked with USPS and other government agencies and the postal worker unions to evaluate whether additional environmental sampling was warranted at facilities that had tested negative based on earlier sampling results. This led to a report issued on August 27, 2004, that concluded that the anthrax risk level for postal workers in the facilities tested, along with the general public served by those facilities was negligible and that no further sampling was warranted. Key factors in the conclusion were the use of anthrax-related cleaning efforts, controls, and work practices at USPS facilities; the nature of sampling performed at facilities known to have processed the source letters; and the passage of two and a half years without additional health concerns (USPS, 2004).

CDC also worked with USPS and public health partners to create guidance for responding to detection of aerosolized *B. anthracis* by Autonomous Detection Systems in the workplace. This guidance, published in CDC's *Morbidity Mortality Weekly Report* in April 2004, describes the arrangements needed to confirm positive signals and how to develop effective response protocols for such signals. The guidance was designed to meet the needs of USPS for their BDS system and to provide a template for use by other organizations deciding to deploy such systems (Meehan, et al., 2004).

Efforts toward improving and validating sampling protocols

CDC believes that full validation of every possible scenario variation would be impractical and could not take the place of scientific judgment and evaluation of the specific event. However, CDC is making efforts to validate components of the detection process.

Comparative studies

As previously described, CDC conducted comparative "side-by-side" studies at the Brentwood (now Curseen/Morris) postal facility to compare the effectiveness of different surface sampling methods for detecting anthrax spores. The studies compared performance of dry swabs, wet swabs, wet wipes, and vacuum methods. The applied research also examined the performance of Polymerase Chain Reaction (PCR) technology in comparison to culture approaches. At the Trenton postal facility, CDC performed "side by side" testing to evaluate the sensitivity of several air sampling methods and filter types. These studies provided important information on the performance of the methods. Results were shared with USPS, EPA, and other investigators and were published in the peer reviewed literature to improve overall assessment capabilities (Sanderson, et al, 2002). This information was utilized at facilities undergoing remediation for characterization and clearance sampling.

<u>Laboratory studies</u>

Since 2001, CDC has learned that sampling materials are different, both in their ability to remove spores from surfaces or to release them during sample processing. For swabs, the two materials with the best recovery are cotton tipped swabs or macrofoam swabs (Rose LJ, et al, 2004). In addition, CDC has confirmed what has been historically known about surface sampling with swabs: pre-moistened swabs work better. Because of the uncontrolled variables in the sampling process the limit of detection may be a range and not an absolute number. Additional study is needed as these results are based on studies of a single laboratory, and validation will require multiple laboratory participation.

LRN enhancements

CDC acknowledges that laboratory analytic capacity was stretched during the 2001 events, especially in regard to laboratories in closest proximity to the unfolding events. Since then, a strategy for the transport and shipping of sample burdens to other competent LRN labs that are distal to the most heavily impacted labs has been formulated. The capacity to perform real-time PCR, especially at the LRN confirmatory Reference level (formerly known as LRN levels B and C laboratories), has also increased dramatically since 2001. Should another bio-terror event occur, the LRN will mobilize a phone bank of LRN representatives to retrieve periodic updates of laboratory capacity and projected sample throughput. In addition, the LRN has made advances in electronic data exchange in order to facilitate the rapid communication of laboratory test results in an emergency situation. .

Collaborative studies

Dugway

Via a September 2002 interagency agreement with the U.S. Army's Dugway Proving Grounds in Utah, CDC is supporting research to improve environmental exposure sampling methods for bio-terrorism response investigations. The study uses three surface concentrations and three air concentrations. These concentrations are expected to allow for estimates of lower limits of detection for the sampling methods. The study will also generate samples for additional EPA testing of QPCR (Quantitative Polymerase Chain Reaction) at an offsite facility.

Lastly, the Dugway test chamber and protocol will support testing of additional agents or their non-pathogenic simulants. Preliminary work was recently completed and testing is now underway to:

a) Determine the efficiency of three surface sampling methods (wet swab, wet wipe, and surface vacuum filter sampling) on two types of surfaces (stainless steel and carpet);

b) Determine the efficiency of three air sampling methods (Andersen single stage impactor, PTFE filters, and gel filters);

c) Determine the overall precision of the methods, encompassing sample collection, sample extraction, and sample analysis;

d) Determine intra-lab variability and sample transport factors; and

e) Determine the additional sampling collection efficiency of passing over a surface multiple times.

Sandia

CDC is collaborating with the Sandia National Laboratories in New Mexico and EPA on a DHS funded effort to evaluate current surface sample and extraction methods. The study will also allow for estimates of the lower limits of detection for the methods. Testing is underway to:

a) Determine the efficiency of three surface sampling methods (wet swab, wet wipe, and surface vacuum filter sampling) on four types of surfaces (2 non-porous - stainless steel and painted wallboard; and 2 porous – carpet and bare concrete);

b) Determine the overall collection efficiency of the methods, encompassing sample collection, sample extraction, and sample analysis; and

c) Determine if collection efficiencies are a function of the concentration of spores on the surface being tested.

Summary

Environmental microbiology and sampling issues are important – they provide tools needed for public health decisions, law enforcement investigations, and evaluation of remediation success. CDC is sponsoring research to fill a number of validation gaps for *B. anthracis*. There are many bio-agents of interest, and interagency collaboration via DHS coordination is important for moving forward to improve our overall methods. CDC plans to review the upcoming GAO report closely, and we will work with DHS, EPA, and other agencies to further address issues identified in the report.

This concludes my testimony. I will be happy to answer any questions.

References

USPS, 2004 Response to the General Accounting Office Recommendations on the Anthrax Attacks of 2001. United States Postal Service, August, 2004. http://www.usps.com/communications/news/security/final_gao.htm page 6

Meehan, P. et. al. 2004. Responding to the Detection of Aerosolized *Bacillus anthracis* by Autonomous Detection Systems in the Workplace. Morbidity and Mortality Weekly Report. April 30, 2004/53 Early Release, 1-11.

Sanderson, W. et. al., 2003. Surface Sampling Methods for *Bacillus anthracis* Spore Contamination. Emerging Infectious Diseases. Vol. 8, No. 10, 1145-1151. October, 2002.

Rose, L. et al. 2004. Swab Materials and *Bacillus anthracis* endospore Recovery from Surfaces. .*Emerg Infect Dis* 2004;10(6):1023

Mr. SHAYS. Thank you, Doctor.

Dr. Schafer.

STATEMENT OF DR. KLAUS SCHAFER

Dr. SCHAFER. Chairman Shays, distinguished members.

Mr. SHAYS. I don't think your mic is on. I have never figured this out. Doctors know so much, but they never know to turn their mics on. There you go.

Dr. SCHAFER. Chairman Shays, distinguished members, I am honored to appear before the subcommittee today.

Mr. SHAYS. Thank you. It is an honor to have you, sir.

Dr. SCHAFER. I am responsible for the oversight of the Chem-Bio Defense Program [CBDP] within the Department of Defense. The CBDP is responsible for all aspects of the Department of Defense's fielding of operational chemical, biological, radiological and nuclear defense capabilities, and the chemical, biological, radiological and nuclear force installation program.

The program has efforts across the acquisition life cycle from very early basic research and development activities, advanced development and the procurement of chemical and biological defense capabilities; finally, the entire life cycle management of these field of capabilities to ensure their quality and support while in the hands of the warfighter.

I am accompanied this afternoon by Dr. David Cullen, who is immediately behind me, from the Joint Program Executive Office for Chemical and Biological Defense. The CBDP has been aggressively engaged in the research and development of biological warfare detection and identification technologies. Among these are technologies geared to rapidly and accurately detect anthrax in environmental and clinical samples.

Prior to September 11, 2001, CBDP efforts had focused exclusively on developing capabilities that would eventually be fielded to their operational military forces. September 11th forced a broadening of the Chem-Bio Defense Program focus to provide capabilities in support of installation for its protection and the emerging homeland defense missions. Many of these technologies are the backbone of today's response system protecting the American public.

In pursuit of these new missions, the CBDP has, and is currently fielding these systems and continuing the development of new capabilities which put a premium on sensitivity and precision in the integration of these technologies into the broader interagency response community.

However, while the end mission has changed, the early research and development of these capabilities is still founded on the same basic tenets used to develop capabilities for the operational force, sound science and laboratory validation of technologies. This is always the first step in the eventual fielding of any capability.

In support of the installation force protection and homeland defense missions, the Chem-Bio Defense Program has developed a total systems approach from directing the sample, the laboratory system for the routine analysis of aerosol samples as well as confirmatory analysis of suspect samples from other sources.

The capability is founded on technologies largely developed and validated in DOD laboratories, such world class laboratories as

USAMRIID and the Naval Medical Research Center, which are, by the way, also recognized as definitive Laboratory Response Network laboratories. Technologies, protocols and procedures developed in these labs, as well as others, are then transitioned into a network of laboratories providing capability to insulation force protection.

This is what the Pentagon Force Protection Agency uses today. The CBDP has instituted an overarching Quality Assurance and Quality Control Program that assures these technologies, protocols and procedures developed and validated in the hands of scientists at DOD labs can and will perform with required precision and accuracy in the hands of field activities.

The QA/QC Program involves not only the required documentation of all procedures and processes, but also continual proficiency testing to ensure that the laboratories are performing equally within the framework designed. The Chem-Bio Defense Program has also continually and aggressively engaged with operational units to assure that decisionmaking and risk assessment is coupled with the correct technical information so that timely and accurate operational decisions can be made.

Finally, we have been and we will continue to coordinate the development of technologies with the requisite policymaking that must go hand in hand to create a proficient and capable system. Within the Department of Defense, we are collaborating with the Assistant Secretaries of Defense for Homeland Defense and Health Affairs so technologies we are developing and fielding can be integrated properly and seamlessly into the medical response community and within the interagency to provide these desperately needed capabilities.

To that end we are collaborating with the Department of Homeland Security and the Department of Health and Human Services in studies aimed at gaining VW collection, detection and identification systems, equivalencies between agencies, and we are developing interagency response frameworks that are so important to protecting the American public.

Subject to your questions, that concludes my remarks.

[The prepared statement of Dr. Schafer follows:]

Statement for the Record of Dr. Klaus Schafer
Deputy Assistant to the Secretary of Defense for Chemical and Biological Defense
Before the House Government Reform Committee
Subcommittee on National Security, Emerging Threats, and International Relations
U.S. House of Representatives
Hearing on "Assessing Anthrax Detection Methods"
April 5, 2005

Mr. Chairman and Distinguished Members, I am honored to appear before your Committee. Good Afternoon. I am Dr. Klaus Schafer, the Deputy Assistant to the Secretary of Defense for Chemical and Biological Defense. I am the Principal Deputy responsible for the oversight of the Chemical and Biological Defense Program (CBDP). The CBDP is responsible for all aspects of the Department of Defense's (DoD) fielding of operational chemical, biological, radiological and nuclear defense capabilities and installation force protection. The program has efforts across the acquisition life cycle, from basic research and development activity, advanced development and procurement of chemical and biological defense capability, and finally, the entire life cycle management of these fielded capabilities to ensure their quality and support while in the hands of the warfighter. I am accompanied this afternoon by Dr. David Cullin, Scientific Director, Joint Program Executive Office for Chemical and Biological Defense.

The CBDP is aggressively engaged in the research and development of biological warfare (BW) detection and identification technologies. Among these are technologies geared to rapidly and accurately detect anthrax in environmental and clinical samples. Prior to September 11, 2001 (9/11), CBDP efforts had focused exclusively on developing capabilities for fielding by the operational military force. 9/11 forced a broadening of

CBDP focus to provide capabilities in support of installation force protection and emerging Homeland Defense missions. Many of these technologies are the backbone of today's response system protecting the American public.

In pursuit of these new missions, the CBDP has and currently is fielding these systems and continuing the development of new capabilities which focus on sensitivity and precision and the integration of these technologies into the broader interagency response community. However, while the end mission has changed, the early research and development of these capabilities still is founded on the same basic tenets used to develop capabilities for the operational force; more specifically sound science, and laboratory validation of technologies. This always is the first step in the eventual fielding of any capability.

In support of Installation Force Protection and Homeland Defense missions, the CBDP has taken a total systems approach for sample collection, the laboratory system for the routine analysis of aerosol samples, as well as confirmatory analysis of suspect samples from other sources. These capabilities are founded on technologies largely developed and validated in world class DoD laboratories , like USAMRIID and the Naval Medical Research Center, which are additionally recognized as definitive Centers for Disease Control and Prevention Laboratory Response Network laboratories. Technologies, protocols, and procedures developed in those labs, as well as others, are then transitioned into a network of laboratories providing capability to installation force protection. The CBDP has instituted an overarching Quality Assurance Quality Control

(QA/QC) program that involves not only the required documentation of all procedures and processes, but also continual proficiency testing to assure that the laboratories are performing equally within the framework designed. Furthermore, the CBDP is aggressively engaged with operational units to assure that decision making and risk assessment is coupled with the correct technical information, so that timely and accurate operational decisions can be made.

Finally, we have and will continue to coordinate the development of technologies, hand in hand with the requisite policy making, to create a proficient and capable system. The CBDP collaborates with the Assistant Secretaries of Defense for Homeland Defense and Health Affairs so that technologies developed under our purview can be integrated properly and seamlessly into the DoD medical response community. Furthermore, we work closely with the interagency to provide these desperately needed capabilities for national biodefense. To that end, we are collaborating with the Department of Homeland Security and Department of Health and Human Services to attain interoperability of BW collection, detection, and identification systems and to develop interagency response frameworks for protection of the American public. Because of DoD's implementation of a rigorous QA/QC program and constant oversight, we can provide assurance that the technologies, protocols, and procedures, developed and validated in the hands of scientists at the DoD labs, can and will perform with the required precision and accuracy in the hands of field operators. DoD is and will always stay committed to achieving the highest standards available to insure that our population is safe.

Subject to your questions, this concludes my opening remarks.

Mr. SHAYS. Thank you. Dr. Schafer, would you mind if we had someone reproduce your remarks? We don't have any written testimony from you.

Dr. SCHAFER. I was told this was oral testimony, and I will be happy to provide written testimony at a later date, if that's OK with the chairman.

Mr. SHAYS. Let me ask you this, just so it doesn't happen again in my subcommittee. My staff said you didn't need written testimony? It is usual practice we require it the day or night before you come to testify.

Dr. SCHAFER. No, sir. I was a late add, so I did not prepare testimony. Through the processes, we couldn't get it cleared in time by OMB.

Mr. SHAYS. Well, I understand that part. What you are saying for the record is that you——

Dr. SCHAFER. This is oral testimony.

Mr. SHAYS. You were told just a while ago that you were testifying and didn't have anything written at the time, is that correct?

Dr. SCHAFER. This is my oral testimony, sir.

Mr. SHAYS. All right. Well, that's what we will have to deal with. I'm sorry, excuse me.

Let me just recognize Jon Porter. Do you have a statement you would like to make or something you would like to say?

Mr. PORTER. Actually, I would like to enter it for the record, Mr. Chairman. I will submit it.

But I would also like to welcome a good friend of mine, Linda Stetzenbach. She is here from environmental studies at the University of Nevada Las Vegas, Harry Reid Center. I will embarrass her for the moment. I think she is on the next panel. Welcome. But I will be submitting my statement. Thank you.

Mr. SHAYS. I thank the gentleman.

Mr. PORTER. Thank you.

[The prepared statement of Hon. Jon C. Porter follows:]

STATEMENT FOR THE RECORD
CONGRESSMAN JON PORTER (R-NV-3)
"ASSESSING ANTHRAX DETECTION METHODS"
April 5, 2005

Mr. Chairman, I would like to thank you for holding this hearing today on Anthrax detection, a vital issue that could potentially affect the livelihood of all Americans. I would also like to thank all of the witnesses for their time today and their expertise in assessing this burgeoning security threat. In particular, I would like to take time to recognize Dr. Linda Stetzenbach, Director of the Microbiology Division of the Harry Reid Center for Environmental Studies at the University of Nevada Las Vegas. I appreciate the time she has taken to present her scientific findings to this panel.

The purpose of this hearing is to examine the present effectiveness of anthrax detection methods. Since the events of September 11, 2001, it was necessary that our nation move from a reactive culture to threats that occurred abroad to one of preemptive strategists when dealing with attacks and potential terrorist threats on our home soil. Therefore, as we analyze the effectiveness of detecting anthrax in closed or open air environments, I am particularly interested in the policy procedures in place to accurately detect this biological threat and in the ability of first responder teams and government agencies to respond.

While an anthrax threat is critical for everyone in the nation, it is especially important that proper detection methods be in place to protect the unique economy inherent to Nevada. A substantial percentage of Nevada's economy stems from tourism and gaming. Therefore it is vital that American and foreign visitors are safe when visiting Northern Nevada or the Las Vegas area in Southern Nevada. The strength of Nevada's economy and the livelihood of many Nevadan families depend on the accuracy of detecting this biological weapon.

Mr. Chairman, again thank you for holding this hearing and I look forward to hearing testimony on this issue.

***

Mr. SHAYS. I thank the gentleman. Let me just, as you stated, ask unanimous consent that all members of the subcommittee be permitted to place an opening statement in the record and that the record remain open for 3 days for that purpose. Without objection, so ordered.

And I will ask for unanimous consent that all witnesses be permitted to include their written statements in the record, and without objection so ordered.

Dr. Schafer, we appreciate your being here. We understand you were told recently you would be testifying. So it is good to have you here. We will just have to proceed through questions to ask you.

Dr. SCHAFER. Thank you, Mr. Chairman.

Mr. SHAYS. Thank you.

Ms. Tulis.

STATEMENT OF DANA TULIS

Ms. TULIS. Thank you. Mr. Chairman and members of the subcommittee, I am Dana Tulis, Deputy Director of the EPA's Office of Emergency Management. My office is responsible for providing national leadership to prevent, prepare for and to respond to human health and environmental emergencies, including terrorist events. I appreciate the opportunity to discuss EPA's involvement in the multiagency efforts to detect anthrax during 2001 and GAO's findings in their recent report on anthrax detection.

I would also like to share with you steps we have taken since that time to improve the Nation's ability to detect and respond to anthrax contamination. With me today is Mark Durno, Senior On-Scene Coordinator in EPA's Region 5 and one of EPA's foremost sampling experts.

In responding to the anthrax attacks of 2001, EPA's role at a site generally began after CDC determined the presence of a biological contaminant, in this case anthrax. EPA collected targeted environmental samples at postal facilities in Florida, on Capitol Hill and other nonpostal facilities for the purpose of characterizing the extent of contamination and for subsequent decontamination.

In taking these steps, we used either wet swabs, wet wipes, HEPA vacuum samples or combination of these depending on the site specific circumstances. We did not use dry swabs because we did not believe they were effective.

The GAO report appears to recommend probability sampling over targeted sampling for detecting anthrax contanimation in a building. EPA believes that targeted sampling strategies are valid and necessary for rapidly accessing the likelihood of contamination to ensure that necessary actions can be taken quickly and to protect those potentially exposed. Especially where the source of contamination is known, targeted sampling of services most likely to be contaminated, as determined from incident-specific details such as traffic patterns and air flow within the facility, epidemiological data and forensic information should provide key information to determine whether contamination exists in a facility. Where contamination is known to exist, but the source is unknown, however, use of statistically based sampling, may improve the probability of detecting contamination.

During the anthrax attacks of 2001, there were hundreds of postal facilities potentially contaminated and quick action was needed, therefore we used targeted sampling to minimize people being exposed.

EPA agrees with GAO that there is a critical need for validated sampling and analytical methods, and we are taking a number of steps to address this gap. Although a lot remains to be done, sampling methodologies have improved and are more consistently applied.

EPA is collaborating with other agencies to develop standardized methods and procedures, and anthrax, of course, is one of those contaminants. Techniques are being developed to concentrate samples of chemical and biological contaminants where necessary to facilitate detection at low levels. EPA is also evaluating the performance of emerging and commercially available technologies such as amino acid test kits and water and other methods.

The GAO report notes that extensive sampling efforts constrain available laboratory capacity and it suggests that laboratory capacity can be increased. Unfortunately, it is not that easy to increase laboratory capacity, especially for environmental analyses associated with biological and chemical warfare agents, where capacity is very limited right now or may not exist.

However, when possible, we do look at individual labs to assess whether research capacity is available during time of critical incidence. But there is no environmental laboratory response network analogous to the CDC's laboratory response network at this time.

EPA and other agencies have initiated a number of steps to deal with this problem. Internally, EPA's own Homeland Security Lab Response Work Group was created in October 2002, and we are working closely with the White House's Homeland Security Council, DHS, USDA, DOD, FBI, CDC, FDA, State laboratory directors and a number of associations, including the Public Health Laboratories Association.

We as a work group have developed an on-line Environmental Lab Compendium of State, EPA and some commercial environmental analysis capability for homeland security purposes. We are also working to incorporate the capabilities of other Federal agencies. We have analyzed and mapped current laboratory capacities to determine the national supply of laboratory analyses for chemical, biological and radiological warfare agents, and we are currently analyzing five of the White House Homeland Security Council's scenarios to look at what the need is and therefore we can determine the gap between supply and demand.

We have also established a reserve corps of 79 EPA analysts who can be trained in chemical and biological analyses, and we will be able to assist in meeting surge demand.

CDC and EPA have developed a MOA to work closely together and to leverage the work of the Laboratory Response Network and to define our respective roles in environmental analyses. We have worked closely with the White House's Homeland Security Council to expand the MOA to include all other Federal agencies with existing or developing networks. This MOA, known as the Integrated Consortium of Laboratory Networks, is expected to be signed very soon.

We have already started to meet and DHS has been posting these meetings. Consortium work groups will address consistency in sampling and analytical methods across the agencies. We do appreciate GAO's efforts to improve the Nation's ability to respond more effectively in the future, and we recognize there is a need to validate sampling and analytical methods to improve our tools and to increase national capacity for analyzing environmental samples.

We believe we have taken significant steps in these areas and have greatly benefited by working closely with our colleagues on this panel, and we look forward to continued collaboration.

Mr. Chairman, subcommittee members, this completes my oral statement. I, of course, am open to any questions you may have.

[The prepared statement of Ms. Tulis follows:]

STATEMENT OF DANA TULIS
DEPUTY DIRECTOR, OFFICE OF EMERGENCY MANAGEMENT
U. S. ENVIRONMENTAL PROTECTION AGENCY
BEFORE THE
SUBCOMMITTEE ON NATIONAL SECURITY, EMERGING THREATS, AND
INTERNATIONAL RELATIONS
COMMITTEE ON GOVERNMENT REFORM
U. S. HOUSE OF REPRESENTATIVES

APRIL 5, 2005

Mr. Chairman and members of the Committee, I am Dana Tulis, Deputy Director of the

Office of Emergency Management, within the Office of Solid Waste and Emergency Response at

the Environmental Protection Agency (EPA). My Office is responsible for providing national

leadership to prevent, prepare for, and respond to human health and environmental emergencies,

including terrorist events. We were actively involved in the response to the events of 9/11 and

the subsequent anthrax attacks, and we are working very closely with the Department of

Homeland Security (DHS) and other federal agencies to enhance the Nation's capabilities to

respond to future events.

In addition to playing a substantial role in developing the new National Response Plan,

we are also now staffing up a new, dedicated National Decontamination Team, which will

provide technical expertise for environmental sampling and decontamination of biological,

chemical or radiological weapons of mass destruction. I appreciate the opportunity to discuss

EPA's involvement in the multi-agency efforts to detect anthrax in postal facilities during 2001

and the findings of the Government Accountability Office (GAO) in their recent report on

Anthrax Detection. I would also like to share with you the steps we've taken since that time to

improve the Nation's ability to detect and respond to anthrax contamination.

INTRODUCTION

In responding to the anthrax attacks of 2001, EPA's role at a site generally began after the Centers for Disease Control and Prevention (CDC) determined the presence of a biological contaminant that poses an unacceptable risk to human health. In Florida, EPA collected targeted environmental samples at the U. S. Postal Service (USPS) West Palm Beach Processing and Distribution Center (P&DC), through which the letter or package sent to American Media Incorporated is believed to have passed. These samples were used to characterize the extent of contamination for the purposes of conducting necessary decontamination. We also conducted targeted environmental characterization sampling at five other postal offices downstream of the West Palm Beach facility, also for the purposes of decontamination. EPA did not collect samples at other USPS facilities. We provided technical expertise and advice on the cleanup of a number of contaminated USPS facilities, most notably the Brentwood and Trenton P&DC fumigations, and in some cases, participated in evaluating the effectiveness of decontamination.

On Capitol Hill, we conducted extensive characterization sampling in several buildings to determine how far the contamination had spread and how best to decontaminate the buildings. We also conducted the actual decontamination, and then performed extensive environmental clearance sampling afterwards to make sure that the decontamination was effective.

EPA also convened and chaired the National Coordination Council (NCC), an *ad hoc* subcommittee of the National Response Team (NRT), to facilitate consistency in response across all facilities contaminated with anthrax, and to provide a forum for resolving interagency issues. In addition to EPA and the USPS, other NCC participants included CDC, the Agency for Toxic Substances and Disease Registry (ATSDR), the National Institute of Occupational Safety and

Health (NIOSH), the Occupational Safety and Health Administration (OSHA), and the U.S.

Coast Guard. To document the experience gained during the 2001 anthrax cleanups, the NCC

also produced the NRT's Technical Assistance Document for Anthrax Response. In developing

that document, the NCC decided to include only those methods, techniques, and technologies

that had been used effectively in experience to date, and were appropriate options for use in

future events. Similar to GAO, the NCC determined that experience had shown that dry swabs

were not effective in sampling for anthrax, and as such, their use is not discussed in the

document.

SAMPLING STRATEGIES

The GAO Report appears to recommend probability sampling over targeted sampling for

detecting anthrax contamination in a building. EPA believes that targeted sampling strategies are

valid and necessary for rapidly assessing the likelihood of contamination to ensure that necessary

actions can be taken quickly to protect those potentially exposed. Especially where the source of

contamination is known, targeted sampling of surfaces most likely to be contaminated, as

determined from incident-specific details such as traffic patterns and airflow within the facility,

epidemiological data, and forensic information provided by the Federal Bureau of Investigation

(FBI), should provide key information to determine whether contamination exists in the facility

and whether further characterization sampling and decontamination are necessary. Where

contamination is known to exist, but the source is unknown, use of statistically-based sampling

may improve the probability of detecting contamination.

Statistically-based sampling strategies, in combination with targeted strategies, are also

appropriate for determining the effectiveness of decontamination. Sampling experts from EPA,

CDC, OSHA, and the Department of Army worked together to develop sampling strategies to confirm decontamination effectiveness after the fumigations of most of the facilities for anthrax contamination. Focused sampling was performed in those areas where contamination was discovered prior to decontamination efforts. Biased sampling took place in areas of increased suspicion of previous contamination and those areas expected to be frequented by building personnel in the future. Grid or random sampling was done in the remaining areas of the facility. A totally random sampling plan might not have specified sampling of areas of known previous contamination and thus would not have provided confirmation that these areas were successfully remediated.

During the 2001 anthrax attacks, there were hundreds of postal facilities potentially contaminated, as well as literally thousands of other "white powder" incidents reported over a short period of time, it was impractical to conduct an exhaustive sampling effort at every potential site. It would also have taken far longer to grid out each location, and then collect and analyze the larger number of samples generally needed for probabilistic sampling. Quick action was needed to identify the most likely areas of contamination and take immediate steps to protect the greatest number of people most likely to be exposed.

ENHANCING NATIONAL LABORATORY CAPABILITY

EPA agrees with GAO that there is a critical need for validated sampling and analytical methods, and we are taking a number of steps to address this important gap. Although a lot remains to be done, sampling methodologies have improved and are now more consistently applied. EPA coordinates research in support of the Agency's homeland security mission and collaborates across the federal government in a variety of science and technology areas. As part of this effort, EPA has been working to develop standardized methods and procedures to support emergency responders and decontamination personnel. Anthrax is one of the contaminants of concern that is being addressed.

These standardized methods and procedures include protocols to sample various types of surfaces and liquids to determine if anthrax is present. Techniques are also being developed to concentrate samples of chemical and biological contaminants, where necessary, to facilitate detection at low levels. Analytical methods being evaluated include (but are not limited to) adaptations of Polymerase Chain Reaction (PCR) methods for determining viability and laser-induced breakdown spectroscopy (LIBS) methods for real-time detection and identification of anthrax spores. Traditional culture methods are also being improved.

EPA is actively engaged in testing and evaluating the performance of emerging and commercially available homeland security-related technologies. To date, four immunoassay test kits have been tested and evaluated for their ability to detect and measure anthrax in water. Additional technologies are being evaluated for detection of anthrax and other threat agents in air, in water, and on surfaces.

EPA has established an intra-Agency work group to address the development of clean-up levels for contaminants (including anthrax as a priority). This work group will provide input to the larger Interagency Committee that has been established by the Office of Science and Technology Policy's Subcommittee on Decontamination Standards and Technology (OSTP/SDST). EPA is developing preliminary risk assessment methods and approaches, and collecting data to support these methods and approaches, for use in homeland security applications.

ENHANCING NATIONAL LABORATORY CAPACITY

The GAO Report notes that extensive environmental sampling efforts can strain available laboratory capacity, and it suggests that laboratory capacity can be increased. Unfortunately, it is not that easy to increase lab capacity especially for analyses associated with biological and chemical warfare agents where capacity is very limited or may not exist. However, when possible, individual labs are accessed for surge capacity during time-critical incidents, but there is no environmental laboratory network analogous to the Laboratory Response Network (LRN) at this time. EPA and other Agencies have initiated a number of steps to deal with this important problem.

EPA's Homeland Security Laboratory Response Work Group, with representation from each media program and five of ten EPA regions, was created in October 2002 to identify and address homeland security laboratory issues. Work Group members have directly engaged in discussions with representatives from the White House Homeland Security Council, DHS, the Departments of Agriculture and Defense, FBI, CDC, and the Food and Drug Administration. State laboratory directors and private associations such as the Association of Public Health Laboratories have also been engaged.

During the past two years, the Work Group has developed a number of tangible products as part of a national solution to analyzing large numbers of environmental samples. We have developed an on-line Environmental Lab Compendium of State, EPA, and some commercial environmental analysis capability. We are also working to incorporate the capabilities of other Federal agencies. Based on the Compendium, we have analyzed and mapped current laboratory capacities to determine the national supply of laboratory analyses for chemical, biological, and radiological warfare agents. We are also in the process of analyzing five of the White House

Homeland Security Council's Scenarios to determine the national need and the gap between supply and demand.

The Workgroup has identified 79 lab analysts from across EPA for inclusion in a trained reserve corps for laboratory support and response. The reserve corps will be trained on chemical and biological analyses. Each of the Regions has established regional/state networks for laboratory analyses and we have recently signed an Memorandum of Agreement with FBI to provide forensic analyses.

We have also begun planning for development of a mobile triage prototype for screening unknown samples before they enter a fixed laboratory. This is essential for protecting the health and safety of laboratory employees. With support and funding from DHS, the first two prototype units will be established at the EPA Region 1 Lab and the New York State Dept. of Health Lab in FY 05.

CDC and EPA developed a Memorandum of Understanding (MOU) to leverage the work of the Laboratory Response Network (LRN) and to define roles and responsibilities between EPA and CDC for environmental analyses. EPA and CDC worked closely with the White House Homeland Security Council to expand the MOU to include all other federal agencies with existing or developing networks. The MOU, known as the Integrated Consortium of Laboratory Networks, is currently under final review by all participating agencies, and the official signing ceremony is expected to take place very soon. The Consortium will establish workgroups to address consistency in the use of sampling and analytical methods across the participating agencies in the network. DHS has already hosted two meetings to further these interagency efforts.

<u>CONCLUSION</u>

We appreciate GAO's efforts to look ahead toward improving the Nation's ability to respond more effectively in the future. EPA recognizes the need to validate sampling and analytical methods, to develop new and better tools for doing this important work, and to increase national capacity for analyzing environmental samples. We believe we have taken significant steps in these areas and have greatly benefitted by working closely with our colleagues on this panel. We look forward to continued collaboration in the future.

Mr. SHAYS. Thank you, Ms. Tulis.
Mr. Day.

STATEMENT OF THOMAS G. DAY

Mr. DAY. Good afternoon, Mr. Chairman and members of the subcommittee. I appreciate this opportunity to meet with you today to discuss the recommendations of the Government Accountability Office regarding validation of anthrax detection methods.

As the Federal agency most directly and tragically affected by the anthrax attacks of 2001, the Postal Service fully understands the value of public and employee confidence and test results for the presence of anthrax. This was an issue raised by the Government Accountability Office in connection with the 2003 hearing of this subcommittee.

GAO recommended that the Postal Service work with other agencies and its unions to consider a number of issues related to the testing of 286 facilities in the fall of 2001, of which only 23 tested positive for anthrax. We were asked to: Reassess the risk level for our employees and customers of the facilities that tested negative; reconsider the advisability of retesting those facilities, employing the most effective sampling methods and procedures; and then finally communicate our conclusions along with our rationale to the Postal Service employees and general public.

Following extensive review by a work group that included experts from the Centers for Disease Control and Prevention, the Environmental Protection Agency, the Occupational Safety and Health Administration and our employee unions, it was concluded that no further sampling was warranted for those facilities that tested negative for anthrax spores.

This decision was based on a number of factors. First, there was no new evidence of anthrax disease in postal employees or customers. Second, the Postal Service had instituted new maintenance procedures and modified work practices to reduce the potential for reaerosolization of anthrax spores. Third, that additional testing would not appreciably increase the safety of our facilities for employees or customers.

The Postal Service is continuing to improve its process to protect our employees and our customers from biohazards in the mail. We have installed advanced Biohazard Detection Systems at 107 facilities. Eventually they will be installed at 282 of our key mail processing plants.

To date, the Biohazard Detection System has performed over 550,000 tests involving over 12 billion pieces of mail. To date there have been no false positives.

These automated systems, developed with the cooperation of experts from the Federal Government, the military and the private sector, provide rapid onsite PCR analysis of aerosol samples collected during the earliest stages of mail processing. They allow for quick response to a positive test result, triggering the local integrated emergency management plan, which includes the cessation of operations, facilities shutdown, notification to community first responders, including public health officials who would make any medical decisions regarding potentially exposed employees and customers.

In addition to the Biohazard Detection System, we are also installing a ventilation filtration system designed to contain to release of biohazards as it moves through the mail.

In developing and deploying the Biohazard Detection System, we recognized the need, very real need for standardization of processes to produce reliable, accurate test results in which our stakeholders can have a high level of confidence.

Over the last several years, and as recently as last month, the Postal Service has been the focus of a number of events in which detection systems at other government facilities that receive mail have indicated possible presence of a biohazard. In each of these cases the Postal Service implemented a response plan that involved sampling and testing, operational adjustments and, where appropriate, preventive medical treatment for employees.

Ultimately, investigation and further testing determined that mail was not involved in these incidents and, in fact, that no biohazards were present. The initial positive alerts, however, appear to reflect the varying capabilities of detection equipment as well as sampling and testing protocols relied upon by other agencies.

Based on our experience, we agree with the Government Accountability Office recommendation that there be coordinated interagency efforts to develop standardized processes in connection with sample collection, transportation, extraction and analysis. However, based on our experience, we believe that targeted sampling, rather than the probability sampling recommended by the GAO, represents the most prudent and productive approach for the Postal Service.

We believe probability sampling can be of value as a sampling protocol in response to a random event. However, once mail has been identified as a potential source of contamination, it is no longer random. At that point, logic and responsibility dictate that sampling follow the trail of the mail, permitting us to conduct sampling along the path taken by the suspect mail during processing.

Probability sampling, by its very nature, might not include sampling from a specific location or piece of equipment through which a contaminated piece of mail has moved. This can create the potential for a false negative.

Following last month's incident at the Defense Department's Remote Delivery Facility, we conducted targeted sampling at our Washington, DC, Government Mails Facility, where mail for delivery to the Department of Defense is prepared. Targeted environmental sampling allowed us to focus on the areas and the equipment through which this mail would have moved. While it was found that mail was not involved in the Defense Department, it provides a demonstration of the steps we take when this type of incident occurs.

We quickly implemented a controlled shutdown of the Government Mails Facility. We promptly notified employees and their unions, both at a national and local level. We continued to provide employees and unions with regular information updates until the situation was resolved. We arranged for the distribution of antibiotics to all of the facility's employees on all work shifts, reflecting a decision that was made in conjunction with the Department of Health and Human Services, Centers for Disease Control and the

District of Columbia Department of Public Health. We also promptly accounted for seven employees who were recorded on sick leave during the period of concern to verify that they were not exhibiting symptoms of anthrax.

Considering that incident and others like it, we believe that the recommendations of the GAO, with the sole exception of probability based sampling, would go a long way in minimizing the possibility of similar future incidents. We look forward to working with the Department of Homeland Security and other agencies to implement these recommendations.

Thank you, and I would be delighted to take your questions.

[The prepared statement of Mr. Day follows:]

**TESTIMONY OF
THOMAS G. DAY
VICE PRESIDENT, ENGINEERING
UNITED STATES POSTAL SERVICE
BEFORE THE
U.S. HOUSE OF REPRESENTATIVES
COMMITTEE ON GOVERNMENT REFORM
SUBCOMMITTEE ON NATIONAL SECURITY,
EMERGING THREATS, AND INTERNATIONAL RELATIONS**

APRIL 5, 2005

Good afternoon, Mr. Chairman and members of the Subcommittee. I appreciate this opportunity to meet with you today to discuss the recommendations of the Government Accountability Office regarding validation of anthrax detection methods.

As the federal agency most directly – and tragically – affected by the anthrax attacks of 2001, the Postal Service fully understands the value of public and employee confidence in test results for the presence of anthrax. This was an issue raised by the Government Accountability Office in connection with a 2003 hearing of this Subcommittee.

GAO recommended that the Postal Service work with other agencies and its unions to consider a number of issues related to the testing of 286 facilities in the fall of 2001. Only 23 tested positive for anthrax. We were asked to: reassess the risk level for employees and customers of the facilities that tested negative; reconsider the advisability of retesting those facilities, employing the most effective sampling methods and procedures; and, communicate our conclusions – along with our rationale – to Postal Service employees and the general public.

Following extensive review by a workgroup that included experts from the Centers for Disease Control and Prevention, the Environmental Protection Agency, the Occupational Safety and Health Administration, and our employee unions, it was concluded that no further sampling was warranted for those facilities that tested negative for anthrax spores.

This decision was based on a number of factors. First, there was no new evidence of anthrax disease in postal employees or customers. Second, the Postal Service had instituted new maintenance procedures and modified work practices to reduce the potential for reaerosolization of anthrax spores. Third, that additional testing would not appreciably increase the safety of our facilities for employees or customers.

The Postal Service is continuing to improve its processes to protect our employees and our customers from biohazards in the mail. We have installed advanced biohazard detection systems at 107 facilities. Eventually, they will be installed at 282 of our key mail-processing plants.

To date, the Biohazard Detection System has performed over 550,000 tests involving more than 12 billion pieces of mail. There have been no false positives.

These automated systems, developed with the cooperation of experts from the federal government, the military and the private sector, provide rapid on-site PCR analysis of aerosol samples collected during one of the earliest stages of mail processing. They allow for quick response to a positive test result, triggering the local integrated emergency management plan which including cessation of operations and facility shutdown, notification to community first responders, including local public health officials who would make any medical decisions regarding potentially exposed employees and customers.

In addition to the Biohazard Detection System, we are installing a ventilation and filtration system designed to contain the release of biohazards as mail moves through our processing equipment.

In developing and deploying the Biohazard Detection System, we recognized the very real need for standardization of processes to produce reliable, accurate test results in which our stakeholders can have a high level of confidence.

Over the last several years, and as recently as last month, the Postal Service has been the focus of a number of events in which detection systems at other government facilities that receive mail have indicated the possible presence of a biohazard. In each of these cases, the Postal Service implemented a response plan that involved sampling and testing, operational adjustments and, where appropriate, preventive medical treatment for our employees.

Ultimately, investigation and further testing determined that the mail was not involved in these incidents and, in fact, that no biohazards were present. The initial positive alerts, however, appear to reflect the varying capabilities of detection equipment as well as sampling and testing protocols relied upon by other agencies.

Based on our experience, we agree with the Government Accountability Office's recommendation that there be coordinated interagency efforts to develop standardized processes in connection with sample collection, transportation, extraction and analysis. However – again, based on our experience – we believe that targeted sampling, rather than the probability sampling recommended by GAO, represents the most prudent and productive approach for the Postal Service.

We believe probability sampling can be of value as a sampling protocol in response to a random event. However, once mail has been identified as a potential source of contamination, it is no longer a random event. At that point, logic and responsibility dictate that sampling follow the "trail of the mail," permitting us to conduct sampling along the path taken by the suspect mail during processing.

Probability sampling, by its very nature, might not include sampling from a specific location or piece of equipment through which a contaminated piece of mail has moved. This can create the potential for a "false negative."

Following last month's incident at the Defense Department's Remote Delivery Facility, we conducted targeted sampling at our Washington, DC, Government Mails facility, where mail for delivery to the Defense Department is prepared. Targeted environmental sampling allowed us to focus on the areas and equipment through which this mail would have moved. While it was found that mail was not involved in this incident, it provides a demonstration of the steps we take when this type of incident occurs.

We quickly implemented a controlled shutdown of the Government Mails facility. We promptly notified employees and their unions, both at the national and local level. We continued to provide employees and unions with regular information updates until the situation was resolved. We arranged for the distribution of antibiotics to the all of facility's employees – on all work shifts – reflecting a decision made in conjunction with the Department of Health and Human Services, the Centers for Disease Control and Preventions and the District of Columbia Department of Health. We also promptly accounted for seven employees who were recorded on sick leave during the period of concern to verify that they were not exhibiting symptoms of anthrax.

Considering that incident and others like it, we believe the recommendations of the Government Accountability Office, with sole exception of probability based sampling, would go a long way in minimizing the possibility of similar, future incidents. We look forward to working with the Department of Homeland Security and other agencies to implement those recommendations.

Thank you.

#   #   #   #

Mr. SHAYS. Thank you, Mr. Day.

Dr. Kelley, we saved the best for the last. I say that because you are a true Yankee from Connecticut.

Dr. KELLEY. Yes.

Mr. SHAYS. I don't know how long you have lived in Connecticut though.

Dr. KELLEY. About 6 years.

Mr. SHAYS. About 6 years. Well, welcome to Connecticut. You have the floor. Is your mic on?

Dr. KELLEY. Yes, it is.

Mr. SHAYS. I asked only because you are a doctor.

Dr. KELLEY. I know, we have problems with those things.

STATEMENT OF DR. KATHERINE KELLEY

Dr. KELLEY. Mr. Chairman, members of the subcommittee, thank you for the opportunity to testify on assessing anthrax detection methods.

My name is Dr. Katherine Kelley, and I am here today representing the Association of Public Health Laboratories [APHL]. I am currently the director of the Connecticut Department of Public Health Laboratory. As its name implies, APHL is the association for State and local governmental laboratories that perform testing of public health significance. In the area of terrorism response that includes both human and environmental testing. This work is done through key partnership with the Centers for Disease Control and Prevention and the Federal Bureau of Investigation to provide rapid local response to a biological event, using consistent scientific methods and reagents and nationally accepted evidentiary practices. The structure for this partnership is the Laboratory Response Network [LRN].

The LRN was deployed in response to the mail contamination events post-September 11th. In some States the laboratory role was limited to testing mail distribution centers in support of the early survey to assess the extent of contamination. In other States, such as Connecticut, the laboratory participated in the diagnosis of infected people and clinical investigations to find the source of their infection and environmental investigations of the postal distribution system as a possible source of anthrax and in the environmental cleanup and clearance of contaminated sites.

All this work was carried out under the direction of a joint command center made up of experts from CDC, the Environmental Protection Agency, National Institutes of Occupational Safety and Health, U.S. Postal Service and APHL, and we drew on outside experts as needed.

APHL agrees with the recommendations of the GAO report under consideration today. There continues to be a need for agreed upon, validated methods for clinical specimens and environmental samples that may be encountered in any kind of a threat event.

However, 4 years after these events, it is easy to overlook the highly charged, complex situation of that moment in this Nation's history. I would like to use our experience in Connecticut as an example.

The Connecticut Department of Public Health received CDC funding to build a response laboratory capacity for weapons of mass destruction bioagents. The working hypothesis at that time was that the LRN would be responding to human outbreaks caused by biothreat agents and that most, if not all, of the testing would be of human clinical specimens.

As a followup to the anthrax letter sent to Congress, our laboratory assisted USPS in an assessment of three postal distribution centers in Connecticut. On November 11, 2001, our laboratory tested 53 samples from the Wallingford USPS distribution center as part of the assessment of the facilities that might have been contaminated by the Daschle or Leahy letters.

All samples tested negative. But the machine that processed the mail at Oxford and Seymour wasn't sampled. On November 19th a local hospital contacted the Connecticut State Health State Department to report a suspected anthrax case in an elderly woman from Oxford, CT. Blood culture specimens were transported to our laboratory from the patient, and they tested positive for anthrax using LRN methods. CDC and the FBI were notified immediately. On November 20th, CDC retested the specimens and confirmed anthrax.

Assuming that this was the index case of a potential anthrax outbreak, CDC was asked to provide assistance and a team of epidemiologists was dispatched to Connecticut. In the interim, the FBI and Connecticut State police secured the patient's home.

Over the course of the next few weeks, CDC and State epidemiologists collected samples from all locations the patient had visited prior to her illness and also from every part of her home. The DPH Laboratory tested them all, and they were all negative for the anthrax Bacillus.

One of the CDC epidemiologists was familiar with the USPS bar code system for tracking first class mail. This data were reviewed to see if any mail coming into close proximity to the Daschle or Leahy letters had gone to Oxford or Seymour. One such letter was identified and retrieved for testing. It was positive for anthrax spores even after repeated sampling. This link to the anthrax positive mail directed the investigation to the Wallingford postal distribution center and to a more targeted sampling of the machines that process mail to the Oxford-Seymour route.

Mr. SHAYS. Your 5 minutes are up.

Dr. KELLEY. Yes, OK. To this day there hasn't been a direct link made to that case, but we do believe that the patient was very fragile and that cross-contaminated mail was probably the source of her infection.

As I indicated at the start of my testimony, we agree with the recommendations of the GAO report. However, I would be remiss if I did not mention the challenges associated with the response to chemical terror events.

Federal funding has improved the availability of public health labs to measure chemical substances in people exposed to a toxin. In fact, we drilled that yesterday. There is still, however, much work to be done to increase the capability of public health laboratories to be able to address local events in terms of environmental testing.

[The prepared statement of Dr. Kelley follows:]

Statement By

Dr. Katherine Kelley

President-Elect, Association of Public Health Laboratories

Director of Public Health Laboratories

Connecticut Department of Public Health

On

Assessing Anthrax Detection Methods

Before the Committee on Government Reform,
Subcommittee on National Security, Emerging Threats, and
International Relations,
United States House of Representatives

April 5, 2005

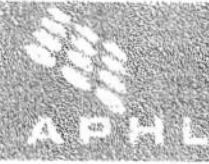

Association of Public Health Laboratories
2025 M Street, NW Suite 550   Phone: 202.822.5227   Web: www.aphl.org
Washington, DC 20036-3320   Fax: 202.887.5098

Mr. Chairman, Members of the Committee, thank you for the opportunity to testify on assessing anthrax detection methods.

My name is Dr. Katherine Kelley and I am here today representing the Association of Public Health Laboratories, APHL. I am currently the Director of the Connecticut Department of Public Health Laboratory. As its name implies, APHL is the association for state and local governmental laboratories that perform testing of public health significance. In the area of terrorism response, that includes both human and environmental testing. This work is done through key partnerships with the Centers for Disease Control and Prevention (CDC) and the Federal Bureau of Investigation (FBI) to provide rapid local response to a biological event using consistent scientific methods and reagents, and nationally-accepted evidentiary practices. The structure for these partnerships is the Laboratory Response Network (LRN).

The LRN was deployed in response to the mail contamination events post-9/11. In some states, the laboratory role was limited to testing of mail distribution centers in support of an early survey to assess the extent of contamination. In other states, such as Connecticut, the laboratory participated in the diagnosis of infected people, in clinical investigations to find the source of their infection, in environmental investigations of the postal distribution system as a possible source of anthrax, and in the environmental clean up and clearance of contaminated sites. All of this work was carried out under the direction of a Joint Command Center made up of experts from CDC, the Environmental Protection Agency (EPA), the National Institute for Occupational Safety and Health (NIOSH), the United States Postal Service (USPS) and APHL, and drew on outside experts as needed.

APHL agrees with the recommendations of the GAO report under consideration today. There continues to be a need for agreed-upon, validated methods for clinical specimens and environmental samples that might be encountered in any kind of terrorist event. However, four years after the events it is easy to overlook the highly-charged, complex situation of that moment in this nation's history. I would like to use our experience in Connecticut as an example. The Connecticut Department of Public Health (DPH) received CDC funding to build laboratory response capacity for Weapons of Mass Destruction (W – M – D) bio-agents. The working hypothesis at the time was that the LRN would be responding to human outbreaks caused by biothreat agents and that most, if not all, of the testing would be of human clinical specimens.

As a follow-up to the anthrax letters sent to Congress, our laboratory assisted USPS in an assessment of three postal distribution centers in Connecticut. On November 11, 2001, our laboratory tested 53 samples from the Wallingford USPS Distribution Center as part of an assessment of facilities that might have been contaminated by the Daschle or Leahy letters. All samples tested negative, but the machine that processed the mail to Oxford and Seymour was not sampled. On November 19, 2001, a local hospital contacted the Connecticut State Health Department to report a suspected anthrax case in an elderly woman from Oxford, CT. Blood culture specimens were transported to the Connecticut

Department of Public Health Laboratory (DPH Laboratory) from Oxford and they tested positive for anthrax using LRN methods. CDC and the FBI were notified immediately. On November 20, 2001, CDC retested the specimens and confirmed anthrax. Assuming that this was the index case of a potential anthrax outbreak, CDC was asked to provide assistance and a team of epidemiologists was dispatched to Connecticut. In the interim the FBI and Connecticut state police secured the patient's home. Over the course of the next few weeks, CDC and state epidemiologists collected samples from all locations that the patient had visited just before she had experienced symptoms and from every part of her home. The DPH laboratory tested them and all were negative for the anthrax bacillus (*Bacillus anthracis.*) One of the CDC epidemiologists was familiar with the USPS barcode system for tracking first class mail. These data were reviewed to see if any mail coming in close proximity to the Daschle or Leahy letters had gone to Oxford or Seymour, Connecticut. One such letter was identified and retrieved for testing. It was positive for anthrax spores even after repeated sampling.

This link to anthrax-positive mail directed the investigation to the Wallingford Postal Distribution Center and to more targeted sampling of the machines that processed mail to the Oxford/Seymour route. In all, the DPH Laboratory tested 465 clinical specimens and over 1,500 environmental samples related to this case. Regardless of the contractor, method of sampling or testing method there were no sites that gave inconsistent results prior to decontamination. This work was performed with continual input from federal experts and utilized lessons that were being learned from the Florida, Washington and New Jersey investigations. There was constant communication between the Joint Command Center and the DPH Laboratory regarding testing capacity, methodology and unusual samples. We were all under intense pressure from our leadership and the press for quick, accurate information. Our laboratory maintained double shifts daily for three months. I am extremely proud of the work done by staff and their dedication to quality science and public health.

To this day no direct link has been made between the Oxford patient and contaminated mail. The assumption is that she may have been exposed to cross-contaminated mail and that this mail had been disposed of prior to her admission to the hospital. It is further assumed that her advanced age and poor health made her more vulnerable to infection.

As I indicated at the start of my testimony, APHL agrees with the recommendations of the GAO report and we continue to press for the development of agreed-upon, validated methods for clinical specimens and environmental samples for any threat agent.

I would be remiss if I did not also mention the challenges associated with a response to a chemical terrorism event.
- Federal funding has improved the ability of public health laboratories to measure chemical substances in people exposed to a toxin. There is still much work to be done to increase the capability and capacity of these laboratories. None of these federal resources have developed any capability or capacity for public health laboratories to accurately measure for chemicals in samples that do not come from

people such as swabs taken from the scene of an incident; clothing from those effected, or even the actual chemical substance.

- There is no comprehensive plan in place today for a response to a chemical terrorism event and there are only three Department of Defense laboratories that could safely and effectively analyze these materials. Currently public health laboratories are not privy to the analytical methods and check standards that have been developed by the Department of Defense, and thus have no ability to perform analyses in a validated and standardized method. In the absence of these materials, public health laboratories will be limited to clinical testing in the response to a chemical event, and will not be able to assist in determining the substance involved in the contamination or its source. This situation is unacceptable, and must be addressed prior to an actual event. Sharing the Department of Defense methods and protocols would be a very good start.

Once again, thank you for the opportunity to testify today and I would be happy to answer any questions.

Mr. SHAYS. Thank you very much.

At this time the Chair will recognize Ms. Norton, give her the gavel for a few minutes, and I will be back in a second.

Ms. NORTON [presiding]. Thank you, Mr. Chairman. My first question has to go to the place where you would, I think if you asked the average person, I think if I asked any of you, if somebody was terrible and treacherous enough to want to do another anthrax attack, what facility of the U.S. Post Office would they go to, and I think you would say, well, they'd go to the facility that handled congressional mail or White House mail. You would say that based on past practice, where two Senators got terribly lethal letters. You would say that based on what we know about al Qaeda and terrorists.

I have to say that I was stunned to learn, and if I am wrong I would like to know that right now, that of these facilities that have gotten the equipment, 107 facilities—and I understand you have to spread them, can't do it all at one time, but 107 facilities, eventually 282 plants, that V Street, where White House mail, congressional mail goes, is not one of the facilities that has these detection systems, is that true?

Mr. DAY. That's correct. As of now, that is a facility that will have it. That facility along with the Curseen-Morris facility, which already has one system, or a modification to the system that we are installing everywhere else. It's a free-standing system. So the V Street facility will have a free-standing system as well the Curseen-Morris facility.

Ms. NORTON. I asked this question not because I think Members of Congress or the White House are entitled to any preference over the average American, but looking at where the priorities for—that I think anybody, even your common sense, even the average layman would say, if you were going to pick, pick 50 places, pick 5 places to start and gave them a description, it does seem to me that at least in the top five, V Street would be there. The mail coming, for example, to the Congress was shut down 3 or 4 days after this until this got straightened out.

So I want to know what are your priorities. How do you decide when this detection equipment will in fact be installed? Is there some method to your madness that escapes me when V Street doesn't have——

Mr. DAY. V Street and the Curseen-Morris facility lack the piece of equipment that the biodetection system is installed on the Advanced Facer-Canceler. So there is a unique application, a free-standing——

Ms. NORTON. So why do the others have it and they don't? First of all, I want to know what your priorities are. First of all, I want to know how you select the order in which facilities get this equipment. Second, I want to know when V Street, which serves the part of U.S. mail most likely to be attacked will, in fact, get such equipment? Those are my questions.

Mr. DAY. The priority has been along the East Coast in the areas that were directly affected. It went onto the Advanced Facer-Canceler System, which is not a system that either the Curseen-Morris or the V Street facility has or will ever have. They don't process that kind of mail. There is a free-standing system that is located at Curseen-Morris. The same system will go into the V Street facility as will additional free-standing systems.

Ms. NORTON. Thank God it is in Curseen-Morris, which everybody should understand is Brentwood, but haven't I gotten an answer from you about how you choose priorities based on the section of the country? OK, so we got the section nailed down pretty clear.

Once you know the section of the country, and there are umpteen places to go, then how do you decide where in fact this equipment is going to go, and when will V Street get equipment? There are people in V Street who were at Brentwood and one of the reasons they wanted to get out of Brentwood is because they couldn't stand to go back in Curseen-Morris and now they learn that—or yet to hear that the equipment isn't in V Street, and I haven't yet heard from you when it will be in V Street.

Mr. DAY. We are working with a contractor to get it deployed in there. I will get back to you with the exact state it will be installed.

Ms. NORTON. I am speaking, I am sure, for the chairman. May I ask that in 30 days you get us a list of your priorities for installation for this equipment and specifically when the equipment will be installed in V Street. Again, this is why I say it is really 2001 all over again.

Let me go to my next question.

Mr. Rhodes. You know, you opened your testimony saying that there are no validated methods for sample collection and analysis, so that agencies, quote, cannot know. As you opened your testimony, I felt like I was hearing someone talk about how we don't have a cure for cancer yet so we cannot know certain things. I mean, is this really rocket science? I mean, what is it?

I don't understand why we don't have any validated methods. Do you mean there doesn't exist any? Do you mean we just don't have any? Would you please clarify why there are no validated methods, 4 years after an anthrax attack. Or perhaps this is more complicated, would you break it down for us so that perhaps the Congress needs to do more to help whoever it is, CDC, EPA, somebody, learn how to validate methods so that they can then be assured that any samples will be as close to valid and what you tell us and what they tell us is possible.

In trying to answer your question about why, I don't know exactly why, other than in the world of chemical, biological, radiological and nuclear countermeasures, biological countermeasures are still considered less important.

Ms. NORTON. Do you think it is a matter that the priority has not been put on finding ways to validate these samples?

Mr. RHODES. Validation methods are well understood. I'm a scientist. Everyone here is a scientist. We know how to validate. It's a matter of is something going to be done. As you've heard from every person here, they've all concurred that validation of methods, they concur with that recommendation.

Let's go back to the 1990's. In the 1990's there were several incidences, actually several hundred incidences of hoax letters being sent through the mail that claimed to have anthrax. As a matter of fact, in the year 2000 alone, the Federal Bureau of Investigation investigated approximately 200 false anthrax letters sent through the mail. At that point in time, methods still weren't validated and people didn't consider biological terror and biothreat to be a high threat.

Since 2001, the fall of 2001, you would think that now that we have five people actually dead from that, 23 injured, seriously injured, that an emphasis on validation of both protocols as well as the techniques, the techniques, the tools, the procedures and the processes, would occur and would be a priority. It hasn't occurred. And I do not know why.

It's not that it's something that isn't understood well by everyone sitting here at the table and other places. It's a matter of are we going to make it a priority; are we going to take the time? Because it's not just enough to say that a dry swab is inappropriate for testing in a particular area. It's taking the entire process of sample collection method—tool, transport, extraction, and analysis—so all of that has to be validated and the inherent errors in the various steps have to be understood so we can have confidence about the answer that comes out at the other end.

Ms. NORTON. Dr. Popovic, I do not understand how you can certify labs if in fact we don't have any understanding in these labs about validating their processes. On what basis are you able to certify the labs that have been certified?

Dr. POPOVIC. I agree with everybody on the panel that validation of a lot of these steps is really important. I would add that there are a lot of steps within this process that have been validated. For example, the protocols for identification and molecular characterization of a number of biothreat agents have existed in 2001 and have been expanded up to this point. At this point, we have added to the laboratory response network 160 protocols to the existing spectrum of what we had since 2001.

The problem here is twofold: One is scientific and one is physical. A lot of these validation studies require two things. One is space that has to be specifically designed. A lot of studies cannot be done with surrogates. They have to be done with the real thing, and so we do need more biosafety level 3 and biosafety level 4 space.

Ms. NORTON. Do you have to have anthrax in order to do it?

Dr. POPOVIC. You can use surrogates for a large number of studies. But you cannot use it for all. So the other thing is you do need diverse scientific expertise. What we are saying here is individual agencies have done some steps of the validation, but as Dr. Tulis has pointed out, this integrated consortium of network laboratories is really a place where all of these individual efforts are now getting to be put together, and we see that as a big umbrella under which really major steps toward validating a lot of these methods are going to be able to take place.

Ms. NORTON. Mr. Chairman, I see you have returned.

Mr. SHAYS. Keep going. The gentlewoman has more time. Let's turn off the clock.

Ms. NORTON. What you last said gave me some hope. Obviously this is something we have had to begun doing after the horrific, tragic anthrax attacks, and we understand that. And you say that this consortium of labs that Ms. Tulis talked about, too, are now apparently getting their act together and what is not an easy process will be taken care of. And I have every confidence that you are doing that.

The problem we have is that in the meantime, these false positives, these false alarms—imagine yourself working in a postal facility today, hearing the testimony you have heard here. Nobody can tell you if it is or if it's not; so if they say it's not, they are not going to believe it's not. It must be terribly anxiety-producing.

I must ask you, even given the complexity of the process you describe, when you think we will get validated testing somewhere, so that we don't have the GAO telling us that there's nowhere—because they say anywhere, there's nowhere anyway—there's no way anywhere, rather, in our country to know, when you get a sample, if it is negative or positive, regardless of what the lab tells you. That is extremely disconcerting for us to hear here, not to mention postal workers who every day have to deal with our mail here.

So I have to ask you, when do you think we will in fact have this validation process underway so that at least the GAO will tell us there is somewhere in America where validated testing goes on?

Dr. POPOVIC. I would like to emphasize once again that the steps for confirmatory identifications have been validated, and those are the steps that are necessary to be linked with the initial signals that come out of various early warning systems such as BioWatch, BioHazard detection systems. Efforts are really underway, and we have already talked with a number of our colleagues on trying to coordinate these initial signals with a proper public health response, which is what you are asking: When can we know that the initial signal is going to be confirmed?

Confirmatory tests can be done within the LRN within the day, within several hours actually, so we are already working on that.

Ms. NORTON. We should remember that this has occurred after this mail has gone and been irradiated, or whatever we call it, and so obviously the chances are low. I do not want to scare everybody. But nevertheless, everybody knows that none of this is perfect. I am concerned that you have not given us a protocol for how you are going to get there and when you are going to get there. And knowing this chairman, I think he is going to want you to be more specific than that. I do not know if Miss Tulis is prepared to be more specific.

But to say we are getting there really is not good enough, particularly since Mr. Rhodes has clarified that it really isn't rocket science. And he has been clear that in fact if the effort is put there, it can be done. And clearly the effort yet has not been focused here. And we are asking for it simply to be focused enough so that, for example, somebody from the government would be able to say in 6 months, by the end of the year, we ought to have a validated testing protocol so that we could then spread to the labs around the country. So is that too much to ask?

Miss Tulis, you didn't have an opportunity to respond to the question.

Ms. TULIS. On the environmental side, we have had a little bit of a problem, because we don't have the analogous laboratory response network, so we've been working the best we can to leverage the existing resources that are out there. In fact we've been having a number of conversations with CDC and worked on this initial memorandum of agreement which now has been expanded to all the Federal agencies. So what we're trying to do is leverage the resources as best we can.

I don't know if I can give you a timeframe today, but I can tell you that on the analytical side, there is a basic compendium, standard and local methods, which we have put together with other agencies, which really is the first step. And the next step, as we are going through right now, is establishing a validation process for those methods.

Again, I cannot give you an exact timeframe because we need to figure out which ones to validate first and how to go through this process. But it is something that is very much right now of being a high priority.

Ms. NORTON. Just bear in mind that our mail is irradiated before it comes here, for good reason, because this is the place of the tragedy; but the mail of most people in the United States is not irradiated so that the clear and present danger posed, as concerned as I am with the targeted facilities of the U.S. Government—let us be clear, the clear and present danger really is the people of the United States who don't have their mail irradiated. So if it goes to some big post office somewhere where there isn't a government facility, my friends, with what you have just testified here, there is a far greater danger to the average American and to the average American postal worker outside of this region than there is to anyone else.

For that reason I believe that the subcommittee has simply got to look into giving you a deadline for focusing on the validation process so—that Mr. Rhodes of the GAO tells us can happen. And remember what his testimony is. Yes, it is not rocket science. No one has given it the focus that would produce validation. Yet that says it all to me. And without validation, I think you are endangering mail systems throughout the United States. And that is on you, and I think you have to do something about it right now.

Thank you, Mr. Chairman.

Mr. SHAYS [presiding]. I thank the gentlewoman.

I was thinking as we were having this hearing, that we have had hearings that go well before September 11, 2001 in which we talked about, in theory, weaponized anthrax. And we said it had no antidote in a sense that where, if you were not protected before, it could kill you. Then we used Cipro, an antibiotic, to deal with it and it appeared to work better than I think we anticipated. So obviously we keep learning things.

I am wrestling with a few things. I get the sense that CDC thinks from a target, and it starts narrowly and works out, and I get the sense that EPA starts broadly and works in. And then I am thinking to myself, well, is one better than the other? It seems to me they both have their role.

But with the facility in Connecticut, we basically identified someone who was not well, an older person, and I am suspecting from that, the conclusion is that the more frail you are, the more vulnerable you become to the anthrax spores.

I am told you can basically put about a million spores in your hand and have clearly weaponized a very fine structure. You could literally hold about a billion. I'm sorry, not a million, about a billion. And then what I have the sense was we did the CDC model, the person, and we targeted where the flow could go. And so there was part of this building that was not checked out. And in the rafters and in the machinery, we then did the EPA model. We then looked at every aspect and found some spores, anthrax spores.

So far, does anyone want to correct me on what I am seeing has happened? Dr. Kelly, is that accurate or not?

Dr. KELLEY. That's pretty much the way it went, right. The Wallingford facility was sampled many, many, many times and from a different perspective, part being the investigation of the case, and then the extent of the problem; and then was it cleaned up sufficiently. So there were quite a few different ideas that were being called on.

Mr. SHAYS. What's amazing to me is that I make the assumption that the elderly woman who was killed in Connecticut wasn't in the facility, yet she was killed by some contact with spores. I make an assumption—and I want to be corrected if I am wrong—that it's likely that some in the postal facility, they were also exposed, but they had the capability to have not been, to ultimately succumb to it.

Were people in the facility given Cipro?

Dr. KELLEY. Yes.

Mr. SHAYS. So the irony here is that if we are using the model that if you didn't die, it must not be there. Once we use Cipro, you might not even be sick; in a sense, we were using a prophylactic that protected some who were in the facility, so the model that you look at, you look at its impact on the folks there. So in one sense, one of our modeling systems couldn't work properly because we introduced Cipro to it.

Dr. KELLEY. The patient also received antibiotic therapy, but——

Mr. SHAYS. It was too late.

Dr. KELLEY. It was too late.

Mr. SHAYS. And she was how old?

Dr. KELLEY. Ninety-four.

Mr. SHAYS. So the bottom line is, though, it's very possible that we had postal workers who were exposed, who either didn't succumb because the exposure was so slight and they were so healthy, or that they were exposed more significantly but they had actually taken an antibiotic that got them through, and we then never knew they were exposed.

Dr. KELLEY. Correct.

Mr. SHAYS. The chairman raised questions about why is DOD given different—and I'm going to raise it in two parts. Dr. Schafer, this is not in any way directed to you, but in the process of trying to find who would testify, it became very real to us that DOD didn't know; and the fact that DOD didn't know was an indication to us that you have a broad—there are a lot of folks involved, and there is no sense of one person being ultimately in charge. Dissuade of me of that view or help me sort out why it's true.

Dr. SCHAFER. Sure, Mr. Chairman. DOD has had well-established processes in place for a long time. I believe after September 11th, many people tried to put things in place, so that may have been a factor. But there was an element of human error that happened in this particular case. But the processes we have in place for verification of results, we never rely on a single test alone, and there is this process that moves, basically moves through the various layers of the lab, with the final element of that being one of the lab response network labs actually doing confirmation. So I think that's why this particular incident looks somewhat different.

But in general we have put processes in place that mirror the CDC processes, are exactly the same thing, and we are part of that network. So I don't view that——

Mr. SHAYS. You used the words "exactly the same" and "part of the network." My view is that you used validated labs and some that were not. I do not know, what is the proper term? Certified and not certified?

Dr. SCHAFER. Well, let me talk about something called the installation protection program. That was the Secretary's decision to bring 200 military installations, start doing environmental sampling in those. And those processes had to be established primarily because of funding constraints and so on. And the labs are different but the processes are exactly the same. So we are no different than the other agencies in that regard. But we do have different requirements, and so there may be differences in that regard.

Mr. SHAYS. I honestly don't quite understand what you're saying. What I hear you saying is in a sense saying, yes, we used labs that weren't certified but were different.

Dr. SCHAFER. In this particular instance, this was a contract let outside the system.

Mr. SHAYS. Right.

Dr. SCHAFER. And so there was an exception and there was human error as well. So it probably looked a lot worse than it really was. But on the other hand, it generated——

Mr. SHAYS. Describe human error to me. I am not asking for a name, but I am asking for human error in what way?

Dr. SCHAFER. Well, we think there was an error introduced in the laboratory that did the procedure. What I would like to do is defer that to the second, the operational side of the questions that you have, because they have all those details.

Mr. SHAYS. So we will leave on the table that there was human error, and you think the second panel will get the answer to that.

Dr. SCHAFER. I believe there was error in the process which generated the false positive.

Mr. SHAYS. Mr. Rhodes, when you hear the question I ask, what is your reaction? Don't tell me you are thinking about the fact that Illinois lost last night. What is your reaction to what we are wrestling with?

Mr. RHODES. Trying to find a single point of contact relative to this question? I think that is the problem everywhere. As you look at our recommendations relative to DHS—and I understand you want to have another hearing where DHS is actually present, but I have to be very clear. You have read DHS's comments. DHS's response to our report is a few pages of explaining why they can't do it, whether they have the charter or not.

Not everybody in government is supposed to look like the Heisman Trophy, you know, pushing away the problem and carrying their own ball. Somebody has to be in charge. You have to be able to come back and say you are the one who is responsible. You now own the problem. That is how we organize validation and that is how we make it a priority.

Mr. SHAYS. Who do you think owns the problem right now?

Mr. RHODES. Everybody.

Mr. SHAYS. And who should own it?

Mr. RHODES. Well, the Department of Homeland Security is our recommendation, that they should be the one who owns it as a Department; but then within each department or agency, someone has to be designated as the owner and you should have the 1–800 number or something: Iamit.gov. That's the location. That's the person.

Mr. SHAYS. One of the problems in this administration, I think, and in this Congress too, I guess, is that there is not the accountability that we need in a lot of things. I think that the failure to hold people accountable for a lot of bad things that are happening in government is seeping through. Nobody is making claim to it, no one wants ownership, and no one is taking responsibility once something goes wrong.

Mr. RHODES. I guess fallout is the wrong term—but the downstream effect is that you can't get good information. For example, you asked were the postal workers put on Cipro, and everyone jumped in and said yes, right away. Wrong. The moment it was found out that it was positive they were put on Cipro.

There was a postal carrier who delivered a 94-year-old asthmatic shut-in's mail that killed her. His bag was contaminated. His vehicle was contaminated. No one knew it. So once everybody found out that it was positive, then, yes, they were put on Cipro.

As somebody who was in the Hart Building the day that it was contaminated, yes, I was put on Cipro, but that was a very, very straightforward event: Open the letter. It falls on the floor. We all go get our Cipro.

Mr. SHAYS. Let me just understand the concept of validation. We are not sure that we really have a good process in place, correct? Let me back up and say it's very difficult to detect anthrax, would everyone agree? I mean, it costs millions and millions of dollars, because we are in a huge building and we are looking for a few spores that you cannot even see.

Mr. RHODES. And let me extend this, when you say a few spores. If we are talking about your constituent who was a customer at Wallingford, as you've heard, no anthrax detected. There's anthrax in the neighbor's mail, there's anthrax in the postal carrier's vehicle, but no one found in all the sampling that was done in her home, no one found anything.

So if I design a detection system for the lethal dose, 50 percent of 10,000 spores, what we have found in the fall of 2001 is the lethal dose, one, which is an immeasurable amount. She may have completely inhaled all of it, and now we're talking about less than 100 spores. You made the point, a billion spores in the palm of your hand. That's small potatoes. Multiple trillions of spores can be held in your hand if it is weaponized well enough.

Mr. SHAYS. I am an impressionable person, and I may say that at some meeting. Your testimony is that where I said a billion, you're saying you could literally hold trillions of spores.

Mr. RHODES. Absolutely. You can hold trillions of spores in your hand if we're talking 1 to 5 micron with no electrostatic charge and all the rest of that. If we have milled it down to that level, of course, you can hold trillions of it. You can have trillions per gram, depending on the concentrate. So billion is a big number, but trillion is a bigger number.

Mr. SHAYS. So my conclusion is that it's pretty difficult to locate this stuff in a building where you could have a handful, a trillion spores that go through the system, the air ducts and so on. At one point they were even talking about taking down the Hart Building, and I don't know if that was foolish talk, but they were basically saying that they may not be able to get all that is in this building, they would have to tear it down. Which was an extreme statement, but not so far-fetched given what you have just said.

So having said that, we all acknowledge it's difficult to find these spores and determine it; and what you are saying to me is reminding me that what triggered the investigation the second time in Connecticut was someone died we believe because of anthrax, but we never nailed it, affirmed that she in her person and so on, but that it was in the neighborhood. It was with the carrier. It was with her neighbor and on and on.

Mr. RHODES. Just one clarification on that. That was actually the fourth time that facility was tested.

Mr. SHAYS. Having said that, I came to this hearing thinking this is almost an exercise in futility. It's so difficult. How could you ever be certain? We could do the best test and never be certain, so how can we give something a clean bill of health even if we do what you recommend?

So that is what I am still wrestling with a little bit. Maybe you can help me sort that out. What I am wrestling with is we can never know if the positive is real and if the negative is meaningful, because it may be we just didn't find it.

Mr. RHODES. What you can know through validation of both protocol as well as tools, techniques, etc., is you can understand your confidence interval, who comes back to you and says this building is clean, this building is safe. You can then ask them, how do you know, how well do you know, how much confidence do you have in that answer?

Right now, as you've said and as Ms. Norton has said and as Chairman Davis said, we have a nice mosaic of maybes. And the idea is you're always going to get some confidence interval. But if somebody walks up to you and says I'm 90 percent confident or I'm 40 percent confident or I'm 60 percent confident, now you're able to make a public health decision based on how good the data are.

Mr. SHAYS. OK. I'm going to put it in my words. First off, let me ask you, would anyone here like to make a comment to the dialog that is happened so far? Does anyone want to respond to any question I have asked or make a comment? Anybody disagree with anything I've said or anything anyone else has said?

Mr. DAY. Mr. Chairman, you've just used the case of Mrs. Lundgren. The fourth time through is when the positive was finally found, and it was through the ability to track through the trail of the mail to a specific bin on a specific machine. It was targeted sampling that found it ultimately.

I agree with Mr. Rhodes, there's a level of probability sampling that can be done that will have confidence interval around it. But when you have a known event—and that becomes a critical issue for us, is it a known event, known source, versus a random event, unknown source—targeted sampling, as was the case with what happened with Mrs. Lundgren and when we finally were able to find it in the Wallingford facility, it was targeted sampling that found it.

Mr. SHAYS. But what's interesting to me is had she not died, we never would have known that there was in fact anthrax at that facility. We never would have known it, ever.

What I'm hearing you say about the validated approach is that we are going to know the strengths for the most part and weaknesses of the process.

Mr. RHODES. The limits, the limits of detection.

Mr. SHAYS. Fair enough. And we are going to know some consistency from one place to another to another.

Mr. RHODES. Right, right.

Mr. SHAYS. Let me, before going back to Ms. Norton, let me ask counsel to ask a few questions.

Mr. HALLORAN. Dr. Popovic, you said twice that the CDC testing methodology in the lab has been validated. Is that validation, is it the same for clinical samples as well as environmental samples or is there some difference?

Dr. POPOVIC. I was talking about the methods for identification, confirmatory identification. Those are the methods that are the same regardless of what the source of the organism is. Once you isolate the organism, be it from a clinical sample or from an environmental sample, the procedures and steps to identify what the organism is are the same.

Mr. HALLORAN. So that's the gold standard?

Dr. POPOVIC. Correct.

Mr. HALLORAN. Now, work me back from there. Can you repeat what the gold standard is?

Dr. POPOVIC. Once you have an organism regardless of the source, where it came from, it can come from air, from surfaces, from food, from clinical sample, the procedures to identify that organism and say this is Bacillus anthracis and the procedures that are molecular characterization are gold standard. They have been validated. And those are the methods that are used in the LRN.

Mr. HALLORAN. And once that sample walks in your door, how long does it take to get that validation?

Dr. POPOVIC. It can depend on a type of a sample. For example, if you have a clinical sample——

Mr. HALLORAN. Wait a minute. It didn't depend on the type of sample a second ago.

Dr. POPOVIC. OK. Let me back up a little bit. If you have blood from a patient, you can usually grow the organism within 12 to 24 hours, and within another few hours you can perform all of the tests that are necessary for you to be able to say this is the Bacillus anthracis.

Mr. SHAYS. Can you grow it faster than what would happen naturally within the body? I mean, do you speed up the process?

Dr. POPOVIC. You cannot actually grow it faster than it would normally multiply in the best circumstances. Bacillus anthracis is one of the amazing bugs which actually multiplies fairly quickly.

Mr. SHAYS. You're telling me more than I want to know right now. The point is, though, that is not really much of a help, because in the end, the person who has the blood who has been—not infected, because—well, it's infected—who has been infected would be proceeding just along the same lines as when you discovered it. In other words, they would be getting sicker during that period of time. I'm sorry I went off the subject, but unfortunately I'm chairman so I get to interrupt. Remember your line of questioning.

Let me understand this so I don't leave with a false impression. If you find it in the blood, you will find it fast enough to give them Cipro to help them.

Dr. POPOVIC. It depends when the blood was collected. If the blood was at the beginning of the disease, yes. If the blood was collected when the patient was dying, then no. It really depends at what stage of the patient's disease. The sooner the better.

Mr. SHAYS. Clear your mind of everything I asked you and go back to his questions.

Why don't you start over again?

Mr. HALLORAN. Work me back through the process now in terms of the differentiation between clinical and environmental samples and why there seems to be this either/or choice between targeted sampling and environmental sampling. Is it, let me spray the panel here, is that a mutually exclusive choice? Must we make that choice?

Dr. POPOVIC. Do we have to make a choice with it to do targeted or probabilistic sampling?

Mr. HALLORAN. Right.

Dr. POPOVIC. We don't have to make that choice always. There are situations, such as in outbreak investigations, when you need to have rapid assessment, when you need to be able to make a decision, when you need to be able to within a very short period of time to make that decision, then targeted sampling is really efficient and effective.

Mr. HALLORAN. Right. But wouldn't it make sense at the same time to begin to map out your grid and start sampling on that grid at the same time you are doing your targets, to know the zone of exposure you are going to have to go back to anyway, as they found out in Wallingford 5 months later? Why pick one?

Dr. POPOVIC. There are a lot of issues. Sometimes there is a capacity issue. Can you actually handle thousands and hundreds of specimens when you actually have a fairly good scientific judgment based on epidemiology that this is where you need to look.

Mr. HALLORAN. But you could store them, could you not? Do they keep?

Dr. POPOVIC. You can store samples, that is correct. Samples can be stored.

Ms. TULIS. If I may, grids could miss very small areas of contamination where, if you're targeted, you would know to go there, so you could do a larger sample area.

Dr. POPOVIC. One example is if people are coming into a room and you can actually use the grid and sample all of the areas, but if you sample the doorway, many times your chances of getting something there are probably better than just going all over the room because the concentration of the entrance of—in this case let's talk about bacteria—would be a smaller area that you can focus on.

Mr. HALLORAN. So you said, the chances are. It strikes me either way it is a crap shoot here. Where are the odds better?

Dr. POPOVIC. I'm sorry; I did not hear you.

Mr. HALLORAN. Where are the odds better that you will find what you need to find to be able to make a conclusion with some confidence of what you have found or not found?

Dr. POPOVIC. If you have epidemiological information, if you have assessment of the individual event, then your chances and the odds are better that you will get the results quicker with the targeted sampling.

Mr. HALLORAN. But in the nonspecific event that Mr. Day referred to, when you have a threat or someone says I sent anthrax through there but no one is sick yet, what's your plan?

Dr. POPOVIC. Well, if you look at the nonspecific event and you look at the Wallingford postal facility, the first two samplings were really not targeted, they were sampled as part of the sampling of facilities. But as pointed out, when you actually knew where to look for it and when you focus there, we found it. So there are advantages in different situations. And like I said, for this initial assessment, for making a public health decision, it is really critically important to do this quickly. One of the main reasons is because the period of time within which antimicrobial prophylaxis is going to be effective is short.

Mr. HALLORAN. I understand. Miss Tulis, in your testimony you said, "but there is no environmental laboratory network analogous to the Laboratory Response Network at this time." Should there be?

Ms. TULIS. That's a loaded question. We believe we need to have more capability than we have at this point and we do not have that capability. We're trying to do our best to leverage existing resources. We do need more capacity than we have at this point.

Mr. HALLORAN. But separate environmental from clinical?

Ms. TULIS. It is a separate type of analysis; yes, it is.

Mr. HALLORAN. In what way?

Ms. TULIS. It's different concentrations. Your whole focus is different when you're looking in air versus water versus looking at blood or serum. You're not looking at metabolites. It's a very different set of processes that you use.

Mr. HALLORAN. But in that process you'd still need to get to that point where you could go to the gold standard before you really know; or do you have some confidence in the decision before that?

Ms. TULIS. Generally we come in, once detection has been made, to do the actual decontamination, and that's generally when we're using our environmental sampling.

Mr. HALLORAN. There was another statement to the effect that validation, the concern of validation at the time anyway, was the lack of facilities that could do validation studies. Is there still that capacity constraint or can these studies be done now?

Dr. POPOVIC. I can address that. A lot of work is happening already. I did mention in a lot more detail in my written testimony, CDC has an interagency agreement with the Dugway Proving Grounds where such a chamber for establishing and generating known concentration of spores is available; and it has been available and studies are actually taking place there.

One of the things that is important is, like I said, you really need to use the real thing for a lot of these studies. So there are efforts and there are places where these studies now can be conducted and some of these studies are conducted. Some of the preliminary results from the studies conducted at Dugway will be available in December of this year.

Mr. HALLORAN. Thank you.

Mr. SHAYS. Let me, before letting this panel go, just ask the question of DOD. According to Dr. Kelley's testimony, "There is no comprehensive plan in place today for a response to a chemical terrorism event, and there are only three Department of Defense laboratories that could safely and effectively analyze these materials. Currently, public health laboratories are not privy to the analytical methods and check standards that have been developed by the Department of Defense, and thus have no ability to perform analysis in a validated and standardized method."

She goes on to say, "In the absence of these materials, public health laboratories will be limited to clinical testing in the response to a chemical event and will not be able to assist in determining the substance involved in the contamination or its source."

Is that question pretty clear to you? Can you comment on that?

Dr. SCHAFER. There are more than a couple of facilities capable of doing these procedures, but what I would like to do for the subcommittee is get back to you with the specific breakout of what those are, if that is OK.

Mr. SHAYS. Tell me the impact of what she's saying, just so I make sure you understand and maybe help me understand what she's saying. What's the significance of her point?

Dr. SCHAFER. I presume she's referring to perhaps a response time; that if we have to send all samples to a couple of laboratories, it would take a lot longer. That's probably the only reason.

Mr. SHAYS. Aren't you saying something more than that, Dr. Kelley?

Dr. KELLEY. I am. The Laboratory Response Network that Dr. Popovic and others have talked about is primarily set out for biological agents. And we do have the capacity that recently has been put into the LRN to look for chemical WMD agents in clinical specimens, in human specimens.

But one of the lessons we learned from anthrax is you don't have one without the other. If you have a human exposure, you want to know where that came from and is it cleaned up. So the environmental testing goes hand in hand with the clinical testing. And a lot of these things we've learned are local. They happen quickly and right within our jurisdictions. We currently do not have the ability to——

Mr. SHAYS. "We" being?

Dr. KELLEY. The State public health labs, the LRN labs at the State and local level, to do any kind of testing for a chemical agent to assist with the investigation, or to be the companion piece to a human exposure.

Mr. SHAYS. Do you want to followup?

Dr. SCHAFER. If I could respond to that. We actually do have the ability in 14 laboratories to do this kind of work. And then there is an interagency effort that's ongoing to try to put some processes in place for chemical laboratory network just like we're doing with the other laboratory network.

Mr. SHAYS. But the point is, it's not very clear how that system is working right now?

Dr. SCHAFER. No. Again, Mr. Chairman, I would be happy to get back to you with the very specifics on that.

Mr. HALLORAN. One final question. Mr. Day, the recent detections in this area were not at the USPS facilities; is that correct?

Mr. DAY. No, absolutely not. Since 2001, all of the false-positive events that have occurred in this area have been at other agencies, not with the postal service.

Mr. HALLORAN. And in the 107 facilities where you have these detection devices operating, describe for us—assure us, if you would, of the response plan: when the red light goes on at one of those facilities, when there is an initial positive what happens? Who calls who, who talks to who; does it look like an ordinary process or does it look like the keystone cops?

Mr. DAY. Let me start at a high level. What we did before we ever deployed the equipment was to develop a template for response. We clearly did not want to deploy the equipment and not have a plan for how we would respond. We worked with other Federal agencies, DHS, CDC, OSHA, EPA, even the FBI to get the law enforcement piece into it.

That template is then taken to a local level or local management team working with their supervisory work force as well as the local union and management associations and the local first responders—police, fire, rescue and public health—are all brought in so that everyone knows who is notified and what the response will be.

Mr. HALLORAN. So, unlike in the DOD situation, when a local first responder comes to a postal facility, he or she knows what that equipment is, knows what its capabilities and limitations are, knows what's inside that building.

Mr. DAY. Absolutely. And we need to know it as well, because as you go out to 282 local and State government entities, the capabilities are quite different. So we need to understand from our standpoint what the local first responder is capable of doing. So there is a nationally developed template that every site utilizes, and then we implement that on a local level with agreement with local first responders, so that when the alarm goes off we know who is notified and what the appropriate actions will be.

Mr. HALLORAN. Finally, just one last chance. As I recall, each of your testimonies agreed with the GAO recommendation to pursue validation of the whole process, including possibility sampling; is that correct?

Dr. POPOVIC. No.

Dr. KELLEY. No.

Mr. DAY. No.

Mr. SHAYS. Are you satisfied? They said no.

Mr. HALLORAN. That is their answer.

Mr. SHAYS. It begs the question why. Ms. Norton.

Ms. NORTON. Well, I must say, I had a different question for Mr. Day, but given Mr. Rhodes' testimony, I can understand about targeted sampling. Of course, I'm thinking also about places in the United States where it would be more difficult to know where the anthrax is, but I also recall from his testimony about the time it took, what has to be done, the followup, the days he talked about in Connecticut, weeks and finally months.

And so to hear you all say, nevertheless targeted sampling is best, even given the false alarms and the time delay, probability testing has its drawbacks too. And I am aware that always we have to balance one against the other.

I wonder. I know the targeted sampling is cheaper. I wonder if that has anything to do with it. I wonder if one has to be done to the exclusion of the other, and why we would only be validating for targeted sampling given the experience in Connecticut and elsewhere with delay and false alarms and the rest. And all of you going against the recommendation of the GAO just sort of leaves us in a real quandary as to—with the government all coming down on one side, and without your telling us why you would want to exclude probability sampling, which is the very recommendation of the GAO.

Ms. TULIS. There's a lot of questions, so maybe we can tradeoff here as partners. I don't think we're saying we want to exclude probability sampling.

Ms. NORTON. I thought that was your response to the last question.

Ms. TULIS. As a total, no. For example, when we went back to the Hart Building we did do statistical sampling before we had reoccupancy of letting people come back in.

Ms. NORTON. So you really had to do that, didn't you? You really had to do the probability sampling before you let people back into the Hart Building?

Ms. TULIS. For reoccupancy, not for detection.

Ms. NORTON. We are all going to reoccupy these buildings, so why doesn't that tell you something? Why shouldn't both be done, Ms. Tulis?

Ms. TULIS. Because the concern is that if you're not targeting where your areas of contamination are and you're using statistics, you can actually miss those areas. And we actually have some statistics, if you're interested, that we can give you on the effectiveness of targeting versus statistical.

Ms. NORTON. Somebody tell me why you cannot do both, as you did in Hart?

Dr. POPOVIC. What I think we're saying is that both don't need to be done at the same time, that each one of them has a specific function in a different situation. And that is why we kind of all said no, because we feel that there is a need for these plans, which components need to be validated in which situations to really be made. And we're hopeful that this integrated consortium of networks of laboratories can actually provide guidance for that. We're thinking that the probability sampling can be a useful tool that can be added to targeted sampling, but we're not looking at it as a replacement for targeted sampling.

Ms. NORTON. I think we all need to give Mr. Rhodes the opportunity to respond to this, since it is all of you against one.

Mr. SHAYS. Why the resistance?

Ms. NORTON. Mr. Rhodes, the chairman is asking why the resistance, do you think, to probability?

Mr. RHODES. I think that the point that keeps coming up relative to targeted is that there is an assumption that the people who walk into the facility actually know something.

As a scientist, I know nothing until it's proven to me. The concern that I have about targeting—and I don't view them as being mutually exclusive. I would view targeting as being a weighted probability. And there was some discussion earlier about you can miss things with the grid. Yes, you can miss things if your grid is not fine enough. That's also a function of probabilistic analysis of space and air current and things like that.

For example, you will note in a standard office, the computer screen is an attractive location. The neon lights are an attractive location. The ceiling tile is an attractive location. So is the carpet and things like that. So you may not want to stand exactly in the middle of the room and take a HEPA sample from the middle of the room. That can be a decision that's made.

The point that we're making is that—and I think the reason that there is resistance is that probabilistic sampling is large sample set. There is no way for the current laboratory network to handle the load that would come off of that. It is not going to be as rapid as people would like.

Now, my concern would be rapid is nice but getting the wrong answer faster and to a greater degree of precision is not useful to us. So I think that hearing a uniform statement of yes, we believe in validation; yes, we believe in this; yes, we believe in process; no, we don't believe in probabilistic; I think it's a function of dollars, network, capacity, it's all those things. And what you're probably— probably—hearing is that these are government professionals who are looking at it and saying, I can't get the money, I can't get the priority.

I go back to my original statement about CBRN, the B is a little b, everything else is really important, even though we haven't encountered that. The thing we've encountered is a bio-attack. Nobody set off a nuclear weapon. Nobody has come in and dumped radiological material with dynamite around it, like the Chechens did over in Russia; but the thing that has happened, people have to complain because they can't get the support on it. If we were taking it seriously we wouldn't be having this argument, because B would be a capital B and it would be as important as anything else.

Mr. SHAYS. There is a gentleman behind. Were you sworn in and did you want to make any comment? Did you want to respond to something here? Identify yourself.

Mr. KIEFER. My name is Max Kiefer with the CDC, National Institute for Occupational Safety and Health.

Mr. SHAYS. Give your card to the transcriber when you leave, if you would, please.

Mr. KIEFER. OK. I was very pleased to hear you mention that industrial hygiene as a basic tenet was very important. Targeted sampling, what is also known as worst-case sampling, is a fundamental basic industrial hygiene tenet that is used to help us target where we sample to try and rapidly get information for making public health assessments and decisions rapidly. That is what was done at Wallingford to get information on where the source of contamination was, as the doctor mentioned.

It was targeted sampling that found the contamination in delivery bar code sorter No. 10, and not probabilistic sampling. Probabilistic sampling does have a role, and we certainly recognize that and want to work and we are doing work at CDC with Sandia National Laboratories to explore the use of probabilistic sampling for a characterization sampling, for remediation sampling, where it does have a very prominent role. But certainly, in the onset of an outbreak, it is very critical for us to really find out where the contamination is very quickly so we can target medical prophylaxis to people quickly, and we don't have the time to wait for 4 or 5 days to grid out a facility.

And I'd like to correct something that was mentioned earlier. The high base sampling in Wallingford was not something that was uncovered due to probabilistic sampling or a different sampling strategy. That was found because—later in the course of routine maintenance on the part of the postal service. Because of the contamination found at DBCS No. 10, there was a concern that there might have been aerosolization, and there was examination of the upper structures above DBCS No. 10 because targeted sampling had been found there; and there was knowledge because of what had happened at Brentwood, that there may have been aerosolization there, and that's why the sampling was conducted there.

Ms. NORTON. Mr. Chairman, could I say what I think the problem is just as I derived it from your testimony? It sounds as if targeting sampling is fine if you—for example, if it's positive, you know something. I think what concerns us, as I understand, Mr. Rhodes' testimony, is that if it's negative, you're not sure if it is really negative. It sounds to me that if it's positive, before you let people back in there, it looks like you're going to do all the probability approaches anyway, so that you really do have a two-step process if in fact it is positive for anthrax.

Where I think the problem comes is that if it is negative for anthrax, at least as I understand Mr. Rhodes, you do not know for sure it is negative because you have done no probability sampling. And some of our testimony, sir, about how things were found later, some of the testimony we've heard here about how they could be in the lights or other places, even though they are not where the target says you should go, would leave people who work there with the negative "but perhaps there are spores in that facility" because you have not done probability sampling. If I'm wrong on that I'd be pleased to hear it.

Dr. POPOVIC. I would just like to comment that it is not just the sampling results that, in the initial phase of an investigation, are weighed in to make a decision whether to close the facility or whether to provide antimicrobial prophylaxis, and there's other factors that play into place and those decisions again have to be made.

Ms. NORTON. Like what?

Dr. POPOVIC. There has to be epidemiological evidence. If you actually, for example, know that there were cases associated with postal facilities and you have had sick people in one facility and you have them at the other, you don't necessarily have to wait 2 or 3 days or how long it takes. You can make those decisions. The kinds of exposure that people had. There is a lot of these epidemiologic background information that really plays into place. You can put people on prophylaxis and then come back after a couple of days and decide whether to continue it or not. So those are the instances where time really is of essence.

Ms. NORTON. And you would have done probability sampling by that time.

Again, you all have not convinced me at least that this is not a two-step process. And if you worked in that facility, I bet you would want it to be a two-step process. And all I can tell you is if it was a two-step process in the Senate of the United States, it better be a two-step process everywhere else. We're not going to have disparate treatment. That was one of the great, huge, terrible lessons that came out of the anthrax scare here. People believed, and believe to this day, that Congress was treated differently. If you're going to do that, you're going to have to develop somehow protocol to do it all.

Mr. Chairman, I never did get to ask my question because your staff asked such a good question.

Mr. SHAYS. You will get your chance. But before the transcriber leaves, I was just thinking that this is like my worst nightmare in college when I was taking statistics and probability, and I was watching the transcriber try to concentrate as we talked about this, and I was hoping that she would stay awake during the whole time here, just given my own record in college during that time.

At any rate, we get to stay awake because we get to ask questions. That is one reason we get to ask questions.

Ms. NORTON. And you have to stay awake because you have to answer them.

I have one last question for the panel today. In fairness, I think I should ask this question of you, because I read Mr. Burrus's testimony. He is on the next panel. You know how concerned I am that V Street, the No. 1 target for anybody wanting to use anthrax, does not have the basic bioterrorism equipment that 107 facilities somehow have.

Mr. Chairman, while you were gone, I asked him to get us a priority schedule and get you a priority schedule in the next 30 days.

Mr. SHAYS. Yes, we would like that, why would it take 30 days?

Ms. NORTON. Thank you, Mr. Chairman.

Mr. DAY. Mr. Chairman, I can get you the schedule tomorrow.

Mr. SHAYS. If you would just give it to our committee so we can make sure that Ms. Norton gets it.

Ms. NORTON. Now, if you don't have the biodetection equipment in V Street, even though V Street serves the Congress, the White House—the one place that the terrorists—the Federal agencies, the places where the terrorists want to get. OK.

But I need to hear, because I am going to ask Mr. Burrus this, and I looked at his testimony, and he doesn't have an answer in his testimony, because I suppose it isn't in his control. But he says that he recently visited V Street.

So not only don't we have equipment in V Street, but he says there's an oscillating fan in V Street, and that is precisely what the first thing that the Postal Service did when the Brentwood anthrax scare occurred was to say, shut down the fan. I want to know why—we already know you don't have—and you haven't given me any reason for why they don't have—biodetection in V Street.

But I want to know why there is a fan there, when our experience just a few blocks away in Brentwood says that fans will distribute the anthrax so you shouldn't have a fan going where there is no equipment, where you can't tell where there might be anthrax there at all?

Mr. DAY. The term V Street actually gets used in a generic way. There are two facilities over there. The facility that processes mail that has the automated equipment in it does not have any fans. That's concurrent and follows the national policy. We have a national policy, ever since the events of 2001, that our automated processing equipment—you are not allowed to have fans that direct air flow toward what we call the feed deck where the most likely release would take place, and that's true in V Street. It's not in place near any of that automated equipment.

It's my understanding at the facility across the street, where the trays are simply prepared to go to the irradiation facility which has no air conditioning, has some fans in there. But, again, that is fully in keeping with the national policy. You will find that true throughout the Postal Service, that areas that do not have automated processing equipment have fans; it is true throughout the Postal Service.

Initially in 2001, we shut down all the fans, and the request from many of our employees was to try to relax that policy. And the policy that's remained intact since then is we do not have fans that are directed at the automated equipment. That is the case at V Street as well.

Ms. NORTON. So the fans are directed at what at V Street? There are fans at V Street.

Mr. DAY. Across the street where the mail is prepared.

Ms. NORTON. There are two places at V Street. One has a fan, and one does not. And the one that does have the fan, what happens in the V Street facility that does have a fan?

Mr. DAY. That's what we call our preparation area. They simply are transferring trays of letters, tubs of flats to go into containers to be sent up to the irradiation facility in Bridgeport. You have no individual distribution of the mail; it's not opened up. It's just sent up prepared to go to the facility. So that's deemed a much lower risk, and we see that as reasonable that in those—those employees be allowed to have those fans. Again, consistent with national policy.

Mr. SHAYS. Bridgeport?

Mr. DAY. New Jersey.

Mr. SHAYS. Thank you, I live in Bridgeport, CT and I just wanted to make sure. All right.

All right, is there any response to a question or a comment on the second tier behind the speakers that have been responding.

Any of those of you who stood up that want to set the record straight or want to correct your boss and lose your job or want to amplify what your boss said. I am serious. Just identify yourself, make sure you leave a card with the transcriber.

Dr. SHARMA. Yes. My name is Sushil Sharma, and I work for Keith Rhodes. I want to clarify and set the record straight, with respect to how we articulate the role of the probability versus the targeted sampling. What we are saying is that, eventually, no matter what, whether you find a positive or a negative, you have to do probability sampling.

What do I mean by that? If you have a positive, in order for EPA to do the cleanup, they have to do a probability sampling. If you don't have a positive, you have to offer some assurance to the public that, if anthrax is present, it is below certain detection limits that our meter could not find. Now, what we said in our report is that, at the outset, you decide how many samples and from where you need to collect in order to have that confidence level.

Once you have done that, then we are not saying, don't use your head or judgment. Of course you should. You should first go to those places which you think would be most likely to, under the grand plan. If you don't find there, continue outwards. So we are not saying one versus the other; we think it is a good blending. There is a role for professional judgment, but there are also occasions when judgment does not work, as was the case in the Wallingford facilities.

On the one hand, we hear that time is very critical for public health intervention. But in the case of Wallingford, it wasn't until 3, 4 weeks that anthrax was detected. So there is a chance, in the case of negative results when the source of contamination is not definitive, that you should have—you should work within the grand plan of probability sampling. Thank you.

Mr. SHAYS. Thank you. I was looking at body language with you, Dr. Schafer and Ms. Tulis, as he was talking. Do you disagree with what he said? I mean, it's almost like I was reading. I will tell you what I was thinking: Easy for him to say, but he doesn't have to do it. OK. Was I reading something incorrect in that?

Ms. TULIS. What I was doing is conferring with our sampling expert to verify the information. He can share some information with you if you would like to hear that further.

Mr. SHAYS. Was he sworn in?

Ms. TULIS. Yes, he was.

Mr. SHAYS. Identify yourself and leave a card.

Mr. DURNO. Sir. My name is Mark Durno. I am a Federal on-scene coordinator with the U.S. Environmental Protection Agency.

Basically, with designing sampling approaches to attack any kind of contaminant, be it biological, chemical or whatever, we establish a hypothesis, or a set of objectives. And then our second step is to identify a sample space from which to collect these samples. And in the case of the Postal Service facilities, the sample space was the buildings where the letters originally passed through down to the buildings to which cross-contaminated mail may have passed.

So the initial sample space, including the mail that had then passed down through the subsequent Postal Service facilities, contained a large number of samples. And if statistics were done on this process, I think you would see that the probability was very good that this sampling approach was adequate.

In addition to that, utilizing targeted or judgmental techniques, we have a much, much greater confidence in the results that we see from that. So I will give you a case in point.

At the Hart Building, for which we designed the sampling strategies for characterization, we established both a grid pattern over the entire Hart Building. We also instituted a judgmental or targeted sampling approach. Using those techniques, 23 locations were found to be contaminated or positive with Bacillus anthracis; 22 of those 23 locations were found through judgmental or targeted technique. One location was found by this grid sampling approach, and it just gives more credibility to the idea that this judgmental approach is one of the most important pieces of designing an appropriate data quality objective-based sampling plan.

Mr. SHAYS. Sounds like nonhuman profiling.

Any other comments? We are going to end this panel soon. We are going to begin the evening portion of our program.

Dr. POPOVIC. May I make one comment?

Mr. SHAYS. Yes.

Dr. POPOVIC. I was thinking to put it in terms of human beings and live people. If you come to your physician, and you say I have certain symptoms and whatever, the physician can draw probably 1,000 different lab tests, and we will eventually, after 3 months, when those come from all of the laboratories pinpointed, but the physician also talks to you, and he targeted those after your symptoms.

So if you have symptoms of knee ache, he is not necessarily going to do a brain biopsy. I am exaggerating of course of. But I think it's really important for us to emphasize that all kinds of information that you make when you make decisions about human beings, you actually make when you work in a setting where a bacteria like anthrax or other bacteria are spread all over the place. I just wanted to draw that comparison. I hope it's helpful.

Dr. SCHAFER. Actually, if I could jump on that, I think this is actually the big issue. There are no silver bullets today.

Mr. SHAYS. Right.

Dr. SCHAFER. And I think that's the bottom line. We all know the various sampling techniques, we know how to use them and how to employ them. One is not necessarily better than the other. And at the end of the day, one has to make the decision as to what is the impact of whatever we find on a human being. So the goal here is, no matter what we do, human judgment has to come into the decision process. The end point is we are all here to try to protect our people. That's all I want to say.

Mr. SHAYS. Thank you. Any other comments from anyone?

Ms. NORTON. Mr. Chairman. Could I just put——

Mr. SHAYS. Sure.

Ms. NORTON. The chairman talked about our evening panel. You can see that this is a chairman that doesn't have show hearings. We really learn something, and the only way we can learn it is to have an exchange. Very few hearings I go to where the chairman says, "and does anybody else in the room have anything he wants to say?" But it does help Members of Congress to learn what we ought to do.

Mr. Day, I just want to be clear what I heard, because it seems to me we have gone from bad to worse. We already have established that V Street, where all Federal mail and all White House mail comes, does not have the biodetection equipment. I asked you a question about fans.

As I hear you, you said that in the particular facility we are talking about, there was a fan, but it was really not the facility we ought to be worried about, because this is a facility where workers are dealing with the mail before it has been irradiated and before it is sent to New Jersey for irradiation. What that means—again, I want to hear your explanation, because maybe I have it wrong again—is that these workers are working where there is no air conditioning. So in order for them to work, they have to say, will somebody turn on the fan?

Well, if you turn on the fan and they are handling mail that has not been irradiated, as, for example, occurred when the mail came to the Senate, then, of course, you are really handling dangerous mail. Yes, it hasn't been opened, but as with the Senate mail, some anthrax could easily come through the openings in the envelope. And there you are with the fan on with unirradiated mail in a non-air-conditioned building, and I am supposed to feel that these V Street workers are really OK. I want you to explain why that is not a situation. If anything, that is even worse than the situation across the street where at least they are working with irradiated mail.

Mr. DAY. Again, that's consistent with our national policy. I would gladly go back.

Ms. NORTON. Excuse me, what is our national policy then?

Mr. DAY. Our national policy on fans that we implemented either late 2001 or early 2002 was to not direct fans at the automated equipment where the pinching occurs with the mail that causes it—if a biological threat were in there—to come out. Mail in trays, mail in tubs, is deemed a much, much lower risk. In just picking up a tray, there is nothing about the activity that is going to dislodge it.

Ms. NORTON. Well, of course, this is the same facility through which the anthrax mail came, through these three facilities.

Mr. DAY. Yes, ma'am. I will gladly go back. I will work with the local union. In a large extent, again, in 2001, we shut off all fans. That was our initial reaction. The feedback we got from employees was, is there a reasonable go-between where instead of all fans, what is reasonable in terms of risk?

Ms. NORTON. You are darn right. And the goal is, get some air conditioning in that building where government mail is handled and where anthrax is likely to occur, to be distributed.

Mr. DAY. I can find out about air conditioning, but that has an air flow associated with it as well. That does not mean, if there's a risk there, that it's eliminated.

Ms. NORTON. You have—across the street in V Street and quote, national policy, I take it does not pertain to air conditioning. Look, Mr. Day, you know, I am willing to go with the flow. I know we are trying to get this together, but I am really not willing to hear excuses about Government mail, White House mail, 4 years after September 11th—I'm sorry, after the anthrax scare—does seem to me that everything should be done in that facility to protect workers, because those are the facilities where people died, where workers are most fearful.

And one of the things that I am asking you to do, whatever you do with the national policy everywhere else, is to remember that V Street and Brentwood are indeed where the deaths occurred and are indeed where the targeted mail for any, any terrorist should be if he is really seeking to do harm to us.

And I am asking that the Post Office this summer take steps to air condition that facility. I am asking that V Street be put at the top of whatever lists you have for insulation of biodetection system. I am particularly concerned about these workers, because they are handling irradiated mail possibly with a fan.

Thank you very much, Mr. Chairman.

Mr. SHAYS. Thank you.

Ms. NORTON. Could I get your promise on that, Mr. Day? Excuse me.

Mr. DAY. The equipment for biodetection will be in there. I will find out the specifics about putting air conditioning in the other building. And, again, the policy is about fans that are directed at those pinch points. That is in effect in V Street. We will continue to do that.

Ms. NORTON. We just ask you to use your common sense when it comes to the kind of facility you are dealing with, and we are dealing with a facility that will most likely be the subject of an anthrax attack. If, quote, the national policy doesn't fit as well then please take steps to protect those who are in that facility.

Mr. SHAYS. I think what Ms. Norton is basically saying is that most Members of Congress would believe that this facility more than any other facility is a targeted facility and should be highest on the list. And that's not a reflection of wanting to protect Members of Congress; it's talking about your postal employees. I think you know it. I am just going to say it that way.

Mr. DAY. We understand and concur.

Mr. SHAYS. I think you do. I think all of you have been excellent witnesses, and we thank all of you, and we thank you for your patience. Is there anything that any of you wish we had asked that we didn't ask that you would like to put on the record?

I honestly learned more from that last question. I mean, we had a hearing on terrorism. I asked at the end of a panel and a noted doctor of a major medical magazine before September 11th said, "I want to share my greatest fear." He said his greatest fear is that a small group of dedicated scientists will create an altered biomedical agent that will wipe out humanity as we know it. This was by someone who was a mainstream doctor. That got our attention. That was before September 11th, and there were no cameras, and there were no print media.

So I learned a lot from that last question, is there anything we need to put on record that wasn't? And it also enables me to say that if you leave here saying we should have asked a question we didn't, it's now on your shoulders because I am saying you can answer it. Any question we should have asked and any that you should have answered?

OK. Thank you so much. You have been a wonderful panel. Very patient. We are very grateful to you. We appreciate your dedication to your work and to your country. We particularly thank the lady from Connecticut.

And I am happy there's a Bridgeport, NJ.

Our next panel is Mr. William Burrus, president, American Postal Workers Union, AFL–CIO; Dr. Linda D. Stetzenbach, director of Microbiology Division, Harry Reid Center for Environmental Studies, University of Nevada, Las Vegas; Chief James A. Schwartz, chief, Arlington County Fire Department; Chief Michael P. Neuhard, chief, Fairfax Fire and Rescue Department; Mr. Philip Schaenman, president, Tridata Division of System Planning Corp.; and Mr. John Jester, director, Pentagon Force Protection Agency, Department of Defense.

We will ask you to stay standing, actually, and we are going to swear you all in. So when you get by your seat, we will swear you all in. Thank you all for your patience.

[Witnesses sworn.]

Mr. SHAYS. I would note for the record our witnesses have responded in the affirmative.

Again, we will go with you, Mr. Burrus. We are really going to try to be as close to 5 minutes as you can. I do appreciate this panel's patience. Let me say the advantage of the second panel is you have heard the questions of the first panel, and there may be things you want to depart from your opening statement, if you feel it's been covered, and speak that way. But your full statement will be in the record.

Mr. Burrus.

STATEMENTS OF WILLIAM BURRUS, PRESIDENT, AMERICAN POSTAL WORKERS UNION, AFL–CIO; LINDA D. STETZENBACH, DIRECTOR, MICROBIOLOGY DIVISION, HARRY REID CENTER FOR ENVIRONMENTAL STUDIES, UNIVERSITY OF NEVADA, LAS VEGAS; JAMES H. SCHWARTZ, CHIEF, ARLINGTON COUNTY FIRE DEPARTMENT; MICHAEL P. NEUHARD, CHIEF, FAIRFAX COUNTY FIRE AND RESCUE DEPARTMENT; PHILIP SCHAENMAN, PRESIDENT, TRIDATA DIVISION OF SYSTEM PLANNING CORP.; AND JOHN JESTER, DIRECTOR, PENTAGON FORCE PROTECTION AGENCY, DEPARTMENT OF DEFENSE

STATEMENT OF WILLIAM BURRUS

Mr. BURRUS. Good afternoon. Mr. Chairman, I would like to thank you and the subcommittee members for the opportunity to address the important issues of this hearing. As requested, my testimony will concentrate on the GAO draft report about the anthrax detection methods as well as the impact of the events surrounding the recent anthrax event at the Pentagon mail facilities. The terrible events of September and October 2001 have had a lasting effect on our country, taking the lives and shattering our citizens' security. Much as we evaluate what can be done to prevent such tragedies in the future, we must apply the lessons learned. The fears postal workers harbor about the accuracy of anthrax testing remain, and they will not be overcome until a comprehensive plan of protection and detection is put in place.

I preface these remarks by stating my belief that in the immediate aftermath of the attack, the U.S. Postal Service acted appropriately based on the limited scientific knowledge available. Postal management relied upon the advice of public health officials, and the unions were informed that critical decisions were made. And when presented with the evidence that postal employees had been exposed, managers did not hesitate to close postal facilities. Mistakes were made, but they were honest mistakes. And hopefully, we have learned from them.

However, in the weeks and months that followed, serious errors were made, errors that could have been avoided. Considerable resources had been expended to study anthrax detection methods since the October 21, 2001 incident. The GAO draft report presents a detailed analysis that reflects many of the concerns that we have raised since 2001.

Following the 2001 attack, the Postal Service initiated testing protocol to evaluate all mail processing facilities. The facilities tested negative, but the experience in Wallingford called into question the accuracy of the sampling and the testing protocol. Subsequent tests using a different method, conducted after the death of an elderly woman, revealed the presence of anthrax.

In response to GAO recommendations to reassess postal facilities that previously tested negative, the Postal Service asserted that, because there had been no accidental incidents—additional incidents of anthrax-related illnesses or death, there was little or no risk to postal workers or the public.

Despite our requests, the Postal Service declined to conduct future tests. We strongly disagree with the rationale and the decision not to conduct additional tests. No one can reasonably suggest that our members should serve as the "canaries in the coal mines" of the years past.

The absence of illness or death cannot serve as proof that all is well. The buildings and their contents must be tested and declared free of agents of bioterrorism. APWU concurs with the GAO report that all testing should utilize the best-known practices, and the methods that will provide results that first and foremost is to protect the employees and the public. In those circumstances where nonvalidated processes have been used, we must ask: Are our postal facilities really safe, or could improper sampling and testing methods have missed anthrax? Could unsuspecting employees be exposed at some future date? While the GAO report does not answer these questions, it brings them to the forefront for a thorough examination.

In 2001, the Postal Service was forced to make an emergency decision regarding the type of samplings to be used in postal facilities, whether to dry swab or wet swab. Despite the fact that the scientific community expressed concerns about the efficiency of the dry swab method, that was the method chosen. This choice was accepted by postal public health officials.

However, it was known at the time—and GAO has now confirmed—that dry swab sampling is less efficient than the wet swab method. The USPS advanced a strategy of targeted sampling that proscribed testing the areas that were most likely to be contaminated. This approach, known as "following the mail and monitoring employees," neglects the use of statistical probability. The APWU and GAO reject the premise that following the mail and monitoring employees can serve as a means of determining contamination. This is unacceptable and should not be permitted by the Congress of the United States.

Recent anthrax-related events at the Pentagon mail rooms demonstrate a number of efficiencies in communication. They highlight the absence of standardized and validated testing protocols and expose the lack of coordination in public messages.

These most recent events serve as the poster child for inefficiency. Many accounts of the Pentagon incident indicate that the initial sampling was done March 10th and that a positive result was announced March 14th. Reports also specify that the positive result was confirmed on March 15th. That means there was a lapse of 5 days between the initial sampling and the confirmation results.

If it had been a true positive, postal workers would have been in grave danger. Had a biohazard been present, postal workers would have been exposed for 8 or 9 days before the results of the confirmation test were received. We know from our experience at Brentwood that waiting even a few days to act can result in death.

Other major concerns arise from the most recent incident as well. First, timely notification was not provided by the Department of Defense to the Postal Service. Second, a certified laboratory was not selected. Third, reporting the results took too long, and as a result, postal workers were potentially at risk. It is fortunate that the positive results were false, but these failures cannot be overlooked.

Mr. SHAYS. Mr. Burrus, you have gone now 6½ minutes, so I need you to wrap up.

Mr. BURRUS. I will. Of major concern is the situation at V Street that has been discussed at some length already. I will defer to questions in more depth about this issue, but the use of fans at V Street, sir, are not for the comfort of the employees. Those fans are used for the exhaust of the gases that are generated by the irradiation of the mail. So I would hope we would get into that subject in a little more depth as we go to the questions.

Mr. SHAYS. Sure.

Mr. BURRUS. Let me conclude, I endorse in large part the inclusion of the GAO draft report and hope you will find them useful in initiating a comprehensive and effective program. Thank you for the opportunity to testify, and I will be pleased to answer any questions you may have.

[The prepared statement of Mr. Burrus follows:]

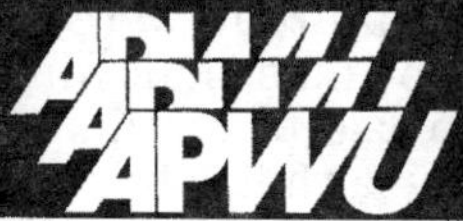

**American Postal
Workers Union, AFL-CIO**
William Burrus, President
1300 L Street, NW
Washington, DC 20005
202/842-4250

Testimony of

**William Burrus, President
American Postal Workers Union, AFL-CIO**

**Improving Confidence in Anthrax Testing:
A Union Perspective**

Before The

**Subcommittee on National Security
U.S. House of Representatives**

April 5, 2005

Good afternoon. I want to thank Subcommittee Chairman Christopher Shays, Ranking Member Dennis Kucinich, and all of the committee members for the opportunity to address the important issues of this hearing. As requested, my testimony will concentrate on the GAO draft report about anthrax detection methods, as well as the impact of the events surrounding the recent anthrax incident at the Pentagon mail facilities.

I am William Burrus, president of the American Postal Workers Union. The APWU is the nation's largest postal union, representing more than 330,000 postal workers in the clerk, maintenance, and motor vehicle crafts.

Postal Workers Continue to Feel the Effects

The terrible events of September and October 2001 had a lasting effect on our country, taking lives and shattering our sense of security. As we evaluate what can be done to prevent such tragedies in the future, we must apply the lessons learned.

Through experience we now know the deadly affect biological agents can have if they are placed in the mail stream. We know that if it is undetected, anthrax can be distributed throughout the country. This knowledge – and the deaths of two of our members – place postal workers on the front lines in the war on terror.

The fears postal workers harbor about the accuracy of anthrax testing following the October 2001 attack remain, and they will not be overcome until a comprehensive plan of detection and protection is put in place.

I preface these remarks by restating my belief that, in the immediate aftermath of the attack, the United States Postal Service acted appropriately based on the limited scientific knowledge available. Postal management relied upon the advice of public health officials; the unions were informed as critical decisions were made, and, when presented with evidence that postal employees had been exposed to anthrax, postal managers did not hesitate to close postal facilities.

Mistakes were made, but they were honest mistakes. Hopefully, we have learned from them.

In the weeks and months that followed, however, serious errors were made – errors that could have been avoided.

Negative Results: True or False

Considerable resources have been expended to study anthrax detection methods since the October 2001 incident. The GAO draft report titled, "Anthrax Detection: Agencies' Validating Detection Methods Would Improve Confidence in Negative Results" presents a detailed analysis that reflects many of the concerns the APWU has raised since the fall of 2001.

Following the October 2001 attacks, the Postal Service initiated a testing protocol to evaluate all mail processing facilities. The facilities tested negative, but the experience in Wallingford, CT, called into question the accuracy of the sampling and testing protocol. Subsequent tests using a different method – conducted after the death of an elderly woman who received mail from the facility – revealed the presence of anthrax.

In response to GAO recommendations to reassess postal facilities that had previously tested negative, the Postal Service asserted that because there had been no additional incidents of anthrax-related illness or death there was little or no risk to postal workers or the public. Despite our request, the Postal Service declined to conduct further tests.

We strongly disagree with the Postal Service's rationale and the decision not to conduct additional tests. No one can reasonably suggest that our members should serve as the "canaries in the coal mines" of years past. The absence of illness or death cannot serve as proof that all is well. The buildings and their contents must be tested and declared free of agents of bioterrorism.

The GAO report underscores the lack of confidence in the testing at postal facilities across the country. Among the many complex issues addressed are the sampling and testing methods used and whether those methods have been validated. The report confirms that many of the concerns the APWU expressed in 2001 were well placed.

APWU concurs with the GAO report that all testing should utilize the best known practices and the methods that will provide results that first and foremost protect employees and the public.

In those circumstances where non-validated processes have been used, we must ask: Are postal facilities really safe, or could improper sampling and testing methods have missed anthrax? Could anthrax be lying dormant? Could unsuspecting employees be exposed at some future date? While the GAO report does not answer these questions, it brings them to the forefront for thorough examination.

In October 2001 the Postal Service was forced to make an emergency decision regarding the type of sampling to be used in postal facilities – whether to use dry-swab or wet-swab sampling. Despite the fact that the scientific community expressed concerns about the efficiency of the dry-swab method, that was the method chosen. This choice was accepted by public health officials. However, it was known at the time – and GAO has now confirmed – that dry-swab sampling is less efficient than the wet-swab method.

The USPS also advanced a strategy of "targeted sampling" that proscribed testing the areas that were most likely to be contaminated. This approach, known as "following the mail and monitoring employees" neglects the use of statistical probability in selecting sampling sites.

The APWU – and the GAO – reject the premise that "following the mail and monitoring employees" can serve as a means of determining contamination. This is unacceptable and should not be permitted by the Congress of the United States.

The GAO report concludes that a coordinated approach is necessary to increase confidence in negative test results. This would include working with agencies and unions to ensure that appropriate validation studies of the overall process are conducted. We concur.

But the GAO report does not go far enough in addressing the importance of the communication of protocols. The unions are a valuable resource in this process and are a primary vehicle for communicating testing procedures and results to employees.

Positive Anthrax Results at the Pentagon

Recent anthrax-related events at the Pentagon mail rooms demonstrate a number of deficiencies in communication; highlight the absence of standardized and validated testing protocols, and expose the lack of coordination in public messages. These most recent events serve as the poster child for inefficiency.

To act effectively, all agencies involved must coordinate the release of information and information must be released immediately. Affected unions must be fully engaged in the process and must understand the rationale for all related decisions. The recent Pentagon incident shows that when unions are not thoroughly involved, the mass media fills the void, often disseminating erroneous or conflicting information.

Media accounts of the Pentagon incident indicate that the initial sampling was done March 10, and that a positive result was announced March 14. Reports also specify that the positive result was confirmed on March 15, 2005. That means there was a lapse of five days between the initial sampling and the confirmatory results. If it had been a true positive, postal workers would have been in grave danger.

If anthrax had been present in mail at the Pentagon, postal employees' exposure would have begun even earlier. That is because government mail undergoes initial processing at the V Street facility in Washington, DC, before it is transported to New Jersey for irradiation. This process can take up to two days. The mail is then returned to the V Street facility to undergo additional sortation prior to being delivered to the Pentagon mail facilities. This can take an additional day. So, prior to being delivered, the mail has been handled by unprotected postal workers for a three- to four-day period.

Had a biohazard been present, postal workers would have been exposed for eight or nine days before the results of confirmatory tests were received. We know from our experience at Brentwood that waiting even a few days to act can result in death.

Other major concerns arise from this most recent incident as well. First, timely notification was not provided by the Department of Defense to the Postal Service that anthrax exposure may have occurred. Second, a certified laboratory was not selected to perform the initial tests. Third, reporting the results took too long and as a result workers were potentially at risk. It is fortunate that the positive results were false and biohazards were not involved. But these failures cannot be overlooked.

Of major concern to the American Postal Workers Union is the alarming fact that postal employees at the V Street facility are not protected by any type of bio-detection system. After the traumatic events of 2001, one would expect that primary consideration would be given to protecting those employees and providing an early warning system.

Instead, all that has been done is to isolate these employees and the government mail sorting operations. If there is real concern that Congress may be a target and that mail may be used as a vehicle of terror, how do we justify withholding protection from the employees on the front line?

Also troubling is what I learned from a recent visit to this facility: in addition to the lack of a bio-detection system, large oscillating fans are being used to circulate air. One of the first precautions taken after the death of two Brentwood workers was to discontinue the use of such fans because of concern that they would circulate contaminated air in the event of future attacks.

There is still a great deal of work to be done and I thank you for doing your part. Postal workers and the mail must be protected. This will help protect the public at large. To accomplish this, we must establish appropriate validating processes and procedures. While we can provide a measure of protection to the members of Congress and their staff through the irradiation of mail, we cannot irradiate employees. They need a different level of protection.

Mr. Chairman and Committee members, I endorse in large part the conclusions of the GAO draft report and I hope you will find them useful in initiating a comprehensive and effective program for bio-hazard protection.

Thank you for the opportunity to testify before your committee. I will be pleased to answer any questions that you may have.

Mr. SHAYS. Thank you for your very helpful statement. Dr. Stetzenbach.

STATEMENT OF LINDA D. STETZENBACH

Dr. STETZENBACH. Good afternoon. I am Linda Stetzenbach, the Director of the Microbiology Division for the Harry Reid Center for Environmental Studies, University of Nevada, Las Vegas, where I have been conducting bioaerosol research for the last 17 years.

I would like to acknowledge Congressman Porter's attendance earlier today, and I know he is very concerned about these issues as well.

Mr. SHAYS. That is Harry Reid of——

Dr. STETZENBACH. The Harry Reid, got us the Senate appropriation to build the building where our research center is located, yes, sir. The university names their buildings after the people that donate the money.

In 1994, I presented results of our laboratory's work on the dispersal of microorganisms into the air at a scientific conference on chemical and biological defense at the Aberdeen Proving Ground in Aberdeen, MD. During a break after my presentation, I was told by one of the attendees that while my data was interesting, anthrax spores would not redistribute into the air once they had settled, and therefore, my data had very little interest for biodefense. This is a——

Mr. SHAYS. How long ago was that?

Dr. STETZENBACH. That was in 1994, sir.

Mr. SHAYS. Interesting.

Dr. STETZENBACH. Later, in June 2001, we published some data using an anthrax simulate in a room-sized environmental chamber that we have had at UNLV since about 1991. Unfortunately, the events in the fall of 2001 demonstrated that dispersal of infectious spores does occur and re-aerosolization does occur. But our earlier data basically was ignored.

Since 2001, it's also acknowledged that monitoring of biothreat agents is problematic due to the lack of standardization and analysis protocols. You heard that with the earlier panel.

For example, there are a variety of sampling methods that have been used by various Government agencies when monitoring for biothreat agents, but the likelihood of success using these methods has not been established. And there are currently no standardized environmental sampling methods for first responders, public health officials, law enforcement agencies and other agencies.

I think it's acknowledged, and you heard earlier, that surface sampling is very useful for determining the presence and concentration of a contaminant, the location where it may have been released, the extent of contamination, forensics and the effect of remediation.

But while swab sampling has a time-honored tradition in the hospital setting from everything from sore throats to wounds, the usefulness of the swab sampling method for sampling buildings is very limited.

One disadvantage is that a large number of samples are generated. For example, tens of thousands of swab samples were collected as a result of the anthrax attacks. And the laboratory response network was simply overwhelmed.

Handling of swabs by emergency personnel responding to an incident is also extremely difficult. Results in our laboratory that we published in 2004 evaluated a Government-developed large area surface sampling method, it's called the BiSKit. It demonstrated the ability to rapidly sample large areas, which translates into better detection and fewer samples. But the swab and the BiSKit are the only two surface sampling methods that have undergone validation testing. Validation testing and the establishment of all protocols used to determine if a biothreat exists in a building is critical.

Therefore, research should be conducted to evaluate currently available and newly developing devices for biological sampling of surfaces. This would provide information on their efficiency of collection and the limits of their capability. You heard that earlier as well.

This information can then be used to determine what device is optimal for what biothreat scenario. An integral part of this research is developing analytical capability through the application of molecular biology methods that enhance the enumeration and characterization of biothreat agents. And molecular biology methods are rapid, sensitive and specific. Unfortunately, there are interferences when you use these methods with environmental samples. They are not clinical samples. They are environmental samples. And simple background dust can give you a false negative.

Therefore, research is needed to minimize the interferences and to optimize analysis of samples from surfaces from the earth and from the air. Also we need to develop standard operating procedures from optimal detection and measurement of biological contaminants. Comprehensive research on these topics would enhance sampling capabilities for the purpose of identification or attribution, while allowing inter-laboratory and interagency comparisons.

There's also serious concerns with assessing the results of bio-aerosol monitoring. We have been focusing today on surfaces, but indoor and outdoor surfaces where air samples are taken is a very real issue. The purposeful dissemination of biothreat agents in enclosed public environments and outdoor facilities that attract the public would potentially result in the exposure of large numbers of individuals.

Therefore, programs utilizing routine monitoring of aerosols has been initiated. Unfortunately, little information is available on the natural background populations of these organisms that are now called biothreat agents. This lack of data has resulted in false positive results with the biowatch system that's currently deployed in selected cities in the United States. A comprehensive survey to determine the levels of naturally occurring biothreat agents would assist decisionmakers when interpreting positive results.

In addition, naturally occurring organisms in the air and on surfaces can affect the ability to discriminate background aerosols from biocontaminants. While some data has been published, the naturally occurring organisms in the types of facilities that may be sites of a purposeful biocontaminant release, such as sports arenas, convention facilities and mass transit, have not been adequately characterized.

The research that I have outlined for you today is vital to provide rapid and accurate information to decisionmakers that are charged with protecting the public health and security of our citizens.

But in closing, I wish to emphasize that universities are an underutilized research resource for much of this research. University scientists have a track record of high quality research on these topics, and they are cost-effective.

In addition, they do not have a vested interest in any method, in any particular protocol, and they can develop and evaluate protocols with an unbiased perspective.

In closing, I would like to thank you for allowing me to come today, and I would be happy to answer any questions.

[The prepared statement of Dr. Stetzenbach follows:]

UNLV

UNIVERSITY OF NEVADA LAS VEGAS

April 7, 2005

Mr. Christopher Shays
Chairman, Subcommittee on National Security

Subject: Subcommittee Hearing April 5, 2005

Thank you for the opportunity to address the National Security, Emerging Threats and International Relations subcommittee hearing that was held on Tuesday, April 5, 2005 at 2:00 pm in Washington DC entitled, "Assessing Anthrax Detection Methods." I hope that the information presented by all the speakers at this hearing will provide your committee with information necessary for decisions regarding sampling for biothreat agents in indoor and outdoor environments.

It was not until I returned to my laboratory in Nevada that I realized a more complete answer was needed to the last question posed to my by the subcommittee. When asked what additional research I thought should be conducted in the studies that are being initiated at the Dugway Proving Ground I should have stated the following:

> While this research is encouraging, it is my understanding that the testing at Dugway is limited to only a few sampling protocols used by the Centers for Disease Prevention and Control. This is too limited and neglects many other sampling methods and protocols that could be useful when attempting to characterize biothreat scenarios in indoor environments. Therefore, additional research is needed.

I have added this statement to my full written statement and have forwarded it to your assistant Kristine McElroy for the record.

Again, thank you for the opportunity to speak at the hearing and for your interest in the issues related to monitoring for biothreat agents.

Should you have any questions please contact me at (702) 895-1419.

Sincerely,

Linda D. Stetzenbach, Ph.D.
Director, Microbiology Division

Harry Reid Center for Environmental Studies
4505 Maryland Parkway • Box 454009 • Las Vegas, Nevada 89154-4009

2

Stetzenbach, L.D.; Univ. Nevada, Las Vegas

Full Statement

Linda D. Stetzenbach, Ph.D.
University of Nevada, Las Vegas

Biothreat agents, such as the spores of *Bacillus anthracis* that cause anthrax, can be efficiently dispersed in aerosols. The spores eventually settle onto surfaces as occurred at the Hart Senate Office building in Washington, D.C. in October 2001. Research has shown that surface-associated biocontaminants can become re-aerosolized, resulting in exposure to building occupants, but detection of airborne and surface-associated biological agents is problematic. Air sampling is useful in determining the concentration and populations of microorganisms in the air at the time samples are collected. Similarly, surface sampling can be used to determine the presence and concentration of biocontaminants on solid and porous surfaces. Surface sampling can provide information on *i*) the location(s) where an agent may have been released, *ii*) the presence and concentration of a contaminant, *iii*) the extent of contamination, *iv*) forensics for law enforcement, and *v*) evaluation of the effectiveness of remediation procedures. However, while a variety of surface sampling methods has been used by various governmental agencies for the detection of biocontaminants, the sampling efficiency and lower detection limits for these sampling methods have not been established, and there are currently no standardized environmental sampling methods. There are no established, validated protocols for first responders, public health officials, law enforcement and other agencies to use when called upon to monitor a building suspected of experiencing a biothreat event. Only two surface sampling methods, the swab and the Biological Sampling Kit (BiSKit), have undergone validation testing. In a study published in 2004 four swab materials were evaluated for the efficiency of recovery of *B. anthracis* from the surface of steel coupons. The authors determined that the greatest recovery of spores was obtained with pre-moistened macrofoam and cotton swabs, and processing by vortexing to remove spores from the swabs. However, the disadvantages of swab sampling include the lack of sensitivity of detection and the large number of samples that can be generated due to the small surface areas sampled. For example, tens of thousands of swab samples were collected following the anthrax attacks and the laboratory response network was overwhelmed with samples. In our laboratory, the surface sampling efficiency of a government-developed large area surface sampling method, the BiSKit, was measured using *B. atrophaeus* (BG), a simulant for *B. anthracis*, and the data were compared with cotton and foam swab-based sampling. Results of this study published in 2004 showed that the primary advantage of the BiSKit was its ability to rapidly sample approximately 1 square yard areas compared to small areas (16 in^2 or 49 in^2), and that the number of bacteria sampled with the BiSKit was 10 times higher. This translates into greater sensitivity of detection and generates fewer samples. Unfortunately, these two studies are the only published data on surface sampling efficiency methods, yet validation and establishment of protocols used to determine if a biothreat exists in a building are vital. Therefore, research should be conducted 1) to evaluate currently available devices for biological sampling of surfaces, 2) to determine their collection efficiencies and sensitivities, 3) to test sample processing methods to enhance retrieval of biothreat agents and to remove inhibitory compounds while minimizing losses of target DNA, and 4) to establish standard operating procedures for optimal detection and measurement of biological contaminants on surfaces. This research would enhance sampling capabilities for the purpose of identification or attribution while allowing inter-laboratory/inter-agency comparison of data. Some validation

Stetzenbach, L.D.; Univ. Nevada, Las Vegas

testing is being conducted in a chamber at the Dugway Proving Ground, Utah. While this is encouraging, it is my understanding that the testing is limited to only a few sampling protocols used by the Centers for Disease Prevention and Control. This is too limited and neglects many other sampling methods and protocols that could be useful when attempting to characterize biothreat scenarios in indoor environments.

In addition, an integral part of monitoring research is developing analytical capability through the application of molecular biology methods that enhance the quantification and characterization of biothreat agents. These methods are rapid, sensitive, and specific, but there are potential interferences resulting from the presence of environmental background material. Researchers have demonstrated that simple house dust can interfere with molecular detection of biocontaminants and that this interference can be overcome, but protocols for sample cleanup have not been established.

Research described above should be performed in a phased approach including both laboratory and bioaerosol release experiments conducted in room-sized experimental chambers. In the first phase, laboratory experiments should be conducted to determine the overall collection efficiency and sensitivity of a variety of currently available surface sampling methods, not just a few selected methods. Representative methods for sampling large areas, small areas and textured surfaces should be tested. Surfaces should include smooth materials (e.g., plastic and painted metal), semi-porous materials (e.g., wood laminate and vinyl tile), and textured surfaces (e.g., fabric and carpet). Sample processing alternatives should be quantitatively evaluated and incorporated into the test protocol to maximize detection of the target organisms. Solutions to interference with molecular detection methods resulting from environmental background (e.g., settled dust) should be investigated by testing sample cleanup methods. The resulting protocols developed from the laboratory experiments should then be validated in research chamber experiments in which bioaerosols are generated, allowed to deposit on test materials, and the surface sampling and analysis is conducted. Innovative and/or newly developed surface sampling methods should be evaluated in laboratory and the research chamber as they are developed. Written Standard Operating Procedures should be developed for the sampling and analysis protocols and a training program for practitioners should be developed and conducted.

There are also serious concerns with assessing the results of bioaerosol monitoring in indoor and outdoor environments. The purposeful dissemination of biocontaminants in enclosed public environments and at outdoor facilities that attract the public would potentially result in the exposure of large numbers of individuals to biothreat agents. However, little information is currently available on the natural background populations of organisms designated as biothreat agents. This lack of data has resulted in false positive results with the Biowatch System that is currently deployed in selected cities in the United States. A comprehensive survey to determine the levels of naturally occurring biothreat microorganisms would assist decision makers when interpreting positive results. In addition, the highly variable composition and concentration of indigenous microorganisms in the air and on surfaces can affect the ability to discriminate background aerosols from biocontaminants. While some data have been published on bioaerosols in agricultural settings, compost facilities, office buildings, schools, and residences, the naturally occurring microorganisms in the types of facilities that may be sites of a purposeful biocontaminant release (e.g., sports arenas, convention facilities, and mass transit system terminals) have not been adequately characterized and interference due to the re-distribution of settled microbial contaminants into the air in these facilities as a result of human activity has not been measured. Therefore, research should be conducted to monitor background populations of airborne microorganisms in a variety of public environments and outdoor facilities, including surface-associated organisms that can be dispersed and interfere with the measurement of purposefully released biocontaminants.

More than 25 scientific papers on bioaerosols, surface sampling, and enhanced detection of microorganisms have been published papers since 1991 by scientists at the University of Nevada, Las Vegas. The following are citations of some of those papers.

Alvarez, A.J., M.P. Buttner, and L.D. Stetzenbach. 1995. PCR for bioaerosol monitoring: sensitivity and environmental interference. Applied and Environmental Microbiology, Vol. 61, pp. 3639-3644.

Buttner, M.P., P. Cruz-Perez, L.D. Stetzenbach, A.K. Klima-Comba, V.L. Stevens, and P.A. Emanuel. 2004. Evaluation of the Biological Sampling Kit (BiSKit) for large-area surface sampling. Applied and Environmental Microbiology, Vol. 70, pp. 7040-7045.

Buttner, M.P., P. Cruz, L.D. Stetzenbach, A.K. Klima-Comba, V.L. Stevens, and T.D. Cronin. 2004. Determination of the efficacy of two building decontamination strategies by surface sampling with culture and quantitative PCR analysis. Applied and Environmental Microbiology, Vol. 70, pp. 4740-4747.

Buttner, M.P., P. Cruz-Perez, and L.D. Stetzenbach. 2001. Enhanced detection of surface-associated bacteria in indoor environments by quantitative PCR. Applied and Environmental Microbiology, Vol. 67(6), pp. 2564-2570.

Buttner, M.P., and L.D. Stetzenbach. 1993. Monitoring of fungal spores in an experimental indoor environment to evaluate sampling methods and the effects of human activity on air sampling. Applied and Environmental Microbiology, Vol. 59, pp. 219-226.

Stetzenbach, L.D., M.P. Buttner, and P. Cruz. 2004. Detection and Enumeration of Airborne Biocontaminants. Current Opinion in Biotechnology, Vol. 15, pp. 170-174.

Stetzenbach, L.D., A.J. Alvarez, and M.P. Buttner. 1996. The Use of Polymerase Chain Reaction (PCR) to Enhance Bioaerosol Monitoring. In D.A. Berg (ed.), Proceedings of the 1994 ERDEC Scientific Conference on Chemical and Biological Defense Research. Aberdeen Proving Ground, MD.

Stetzenbach, L.D.; Univ. Nevada, Las Vegas

<u>Five-Minute Oral Statement</u>

Good afternoon. I am Linda Stetzenbach the Director of the Microbiology Division at the Harry Reid Center for Environmental Studies at the University of Nevada, Las Vegas where I have been conducting research related to airborne and surface-associated microorganisms for more than 17 years.

In 1994 I presented results of our laboratory's work on the dispersal of microorganisms from into the air at a scientific conference on chemical and biological defense research at Aberdeen Proving Ground, Maryland. During a break after my presentation I was told by an attendee that while my data were interesting, anthrax spores would not become airborne once they settled so my research was of little interest to biodefense. Later in June 2001 we published data using an anthrax simulant in a room-sized chamber at out university that has been used for bioaerosol research since 1991. Unfortunately, the events in the fall of 2001 demonstrated the dispersal of infectious spores from letters and postal machinery, and that re-aerosolization of settled microorganisms do occur, and that our data could be useful.

Since 2001, it is also acknowledged that monitoring for biothreat agents is problematic due to the lack of standardized sampling and analysis protocols. For example, a variety of surface sampling methods has been used by various governmental agencies when monitoring for biothreat agents, but the likelihood of success using these sampling methods has not been established, and there are currently no standardized environmental sampling methods for first responders, public health officials, law enforcement and other agencies.

Surface sampling is important for determining the presence and concentration of a contaminant, the location where an agent may have been released, the extent of contamination, forensics, and the effectiveness of remediation procedures.

While swab sampling has a time honored tradition in the hospital setting for everything from sore throats to wounds, the usefulness of this method for sampling buildings is limited. One disadvantage is the large number of samples that can be generated due to the small surface areas that are sampled. For example, tens of thousands of swab samples were collected as a result of the anthrax attacks and the laboratory response network was overwhelmed with samples.

Handling of swabs by emergency personnel responding to a suspected incident is also difficult.

Results in our laboratory of a government-developed large area surface sampler (the BiSKit) demonstrated an ability to rapidly sample a large area, which translates into better detection and fewer samples, but the swab and the BiSKit are the only two surface sampling methods that have undergone validation testing. However, validation and the establishment of protocols used to determine if a biothreat exists in a building are critical.

Therefore, research should be conducted to evaluate currently available and newly developing devices for biological sampling of surfaces. This would provide information on their efficiency of collection and the limits of their capability; information that can be used to determine what device is optimal for which biothreat scenario.

Stetzenbach, L.D.; Univ. Nevada, Las Vegas

An integral part of this research is developing analytical capability through the application of molecular biology methods that enhance the enumeration and characterization of biothreat agents.

Molecular biology methods are rapid, sensitive, and specific, but there are potential interferences resulting from the presence of environmental background material. Simple house dust has been shown to interfere with detection using molecular biology. Therefore, research is needed to minimize interferences, to optimize analysis of airborne and surface samples, and to develop standard operating procedures for optimal detection and measurement of biological contaminants on surfaces. Comprehensive research on these topics would enhance sampling capabilities for the purpose of identification or attribution while allowing inter-laboratory/inter-agency comparison of data.

There are also serious concerns with assessing the results of bioaerosol monitoring in indoor and outdoor environments. The purposeful dissemination of biothreat agents in enclosed public environments and at outdoor facilities that attract the public would potentially result in the exposure of large numbers of individuals. Therefore, programs utilizing routine monitoring of bioaerosols have been initiated. Unfortunately, little information is available on the natural background populations of organisms designated as biothreat agents. This lack of data has resulted in false positive results with the Biowatch System that is currently deployed in selected cities in the United States. A comprehensive survey to determine the levels of naturally occurring biothreat agents would assist decision makers when interpreting positive detection results.

In addition, naturally-occurring microorganisms in the air and on surfaces can affect the ability to discriminate background aerosols from biocontaminants. While some data have been published, the naturally-occurring microorganisms in the types of facilities that may be sites of a purposeful biocontaminant release (such as sports arenas, convention facilities, and mass transit) have not been adequately characterized. Therefore, research should be conducted in a variety of public environments and outdoor facilities to characterize background populations of airborne and surface-associated microorganisms that can be dispersed and interfere with the measurement of purposefully released biocontaminants.

The research that I have outlined for you today is vital to provide rapid and accurate information to decision makers that are charged with protecting the public health and security of our citizens. In closing, I wish to emphasize that universities are an underutilized resource for much of this research. University scientists have a track record for high quality research on these topics and are they are cost effective. In addition, they do not have a vested interest in any particular method and can develop and evaluate protocols with an unbiased perspective.

I would be happy to answer any questions that members of this committee may have. Thank you.

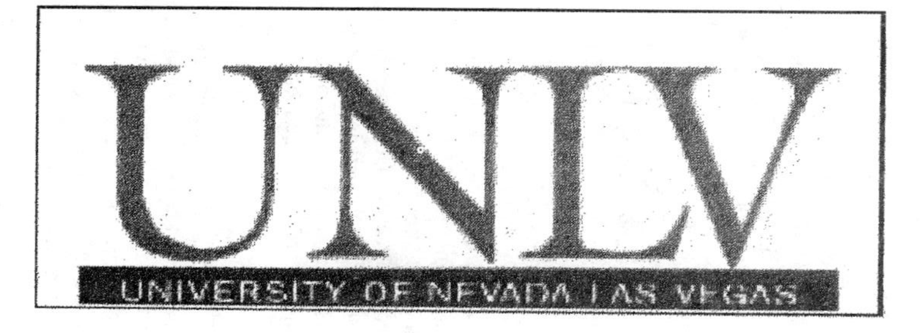

Linda D. Stetzenbach, Ph.D.
Director, Microbiology Division
Harry Reid Center for Environmental Studies
University of Nevada, Las Vegas
STETZENL@UNLV.NEVADA.EDU

1994: studies on the dispersal of settled bacteria from flooring materials in an experimental room due to routine human activity

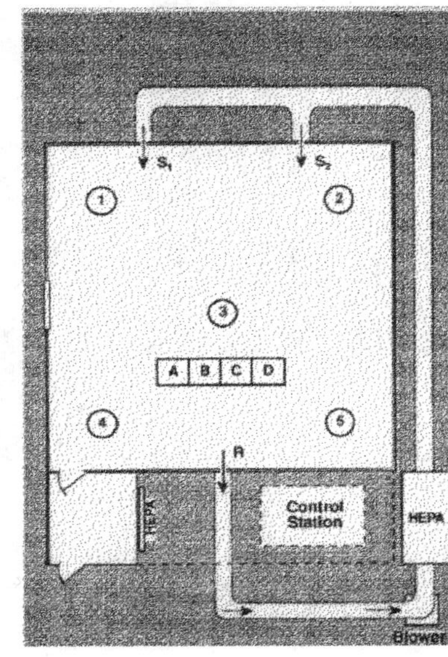

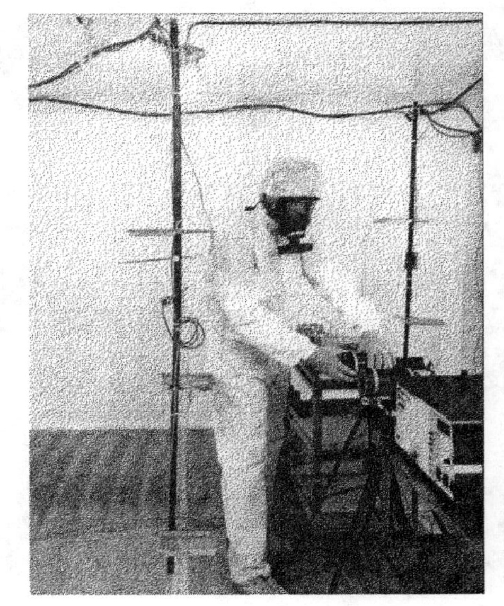

Surface Sampling Methods

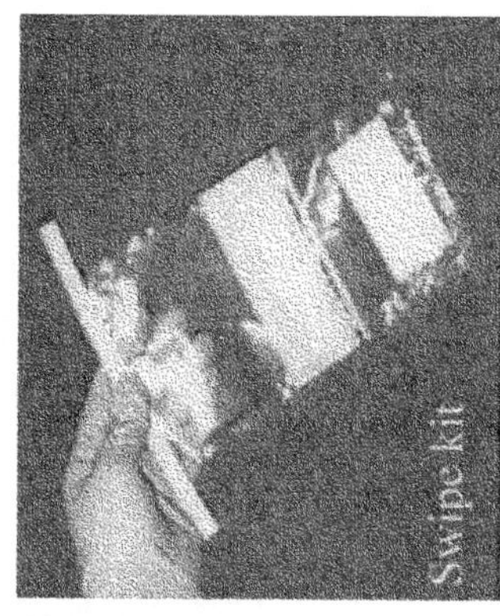

Swipe kit

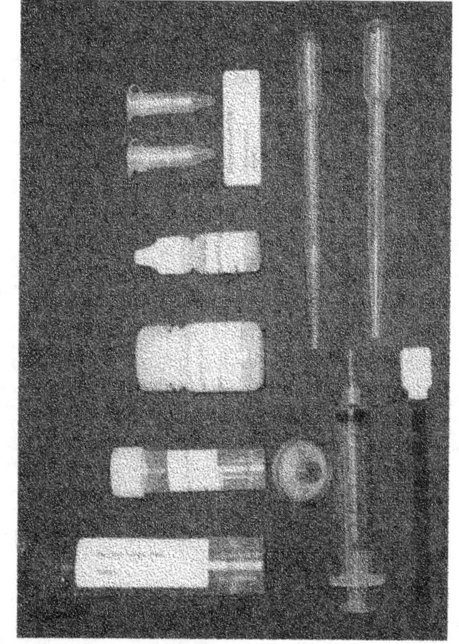

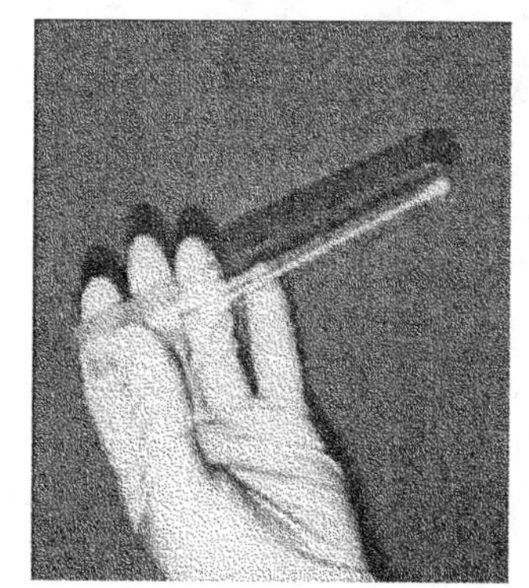

Surface Sampling for Biothreat Agents can Provide Information on:

- Presence and concentration
- Locations where agents were released
- Extent of contamination
- Forensics for law enforcement
- Effectiveness of remediation

Swab Sampling

- Swab sampling
  - sterile cotton swab
  - traditional uses in hospitals
  - numerous samples may overwhelm analytical laboratory

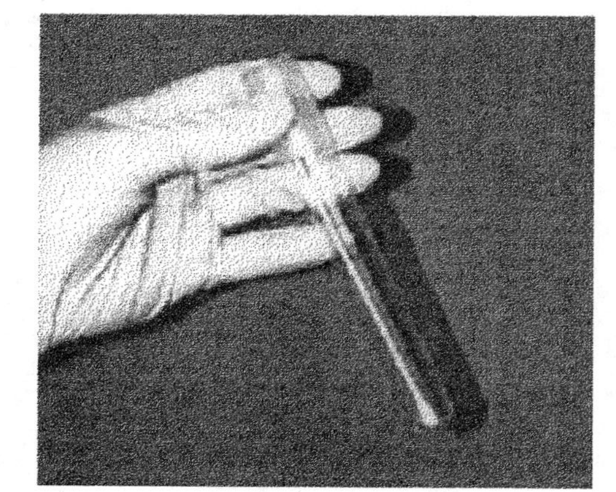

Swab Sampling

- Difficult to manipulate with personnel in protective gear

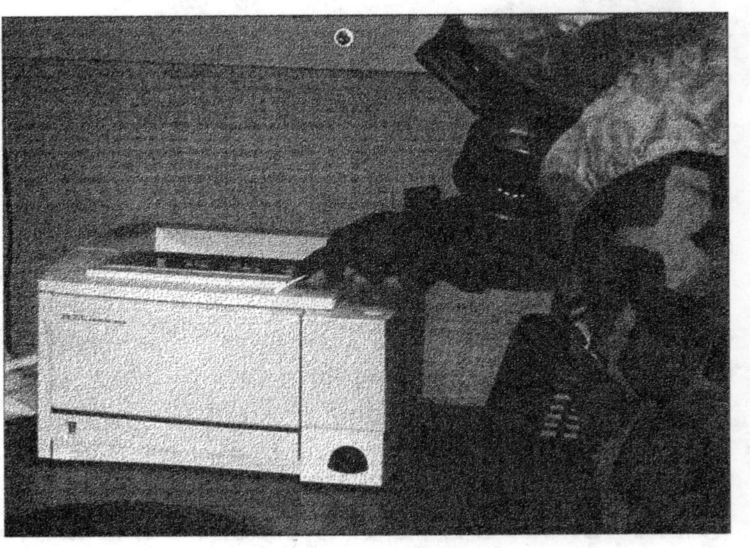

BisKit - large area surface sampling

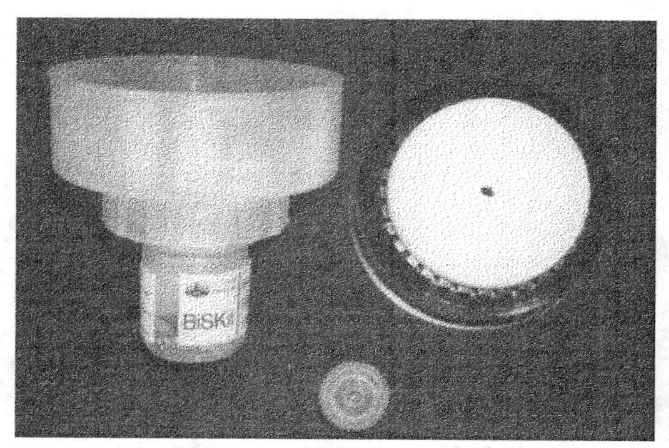

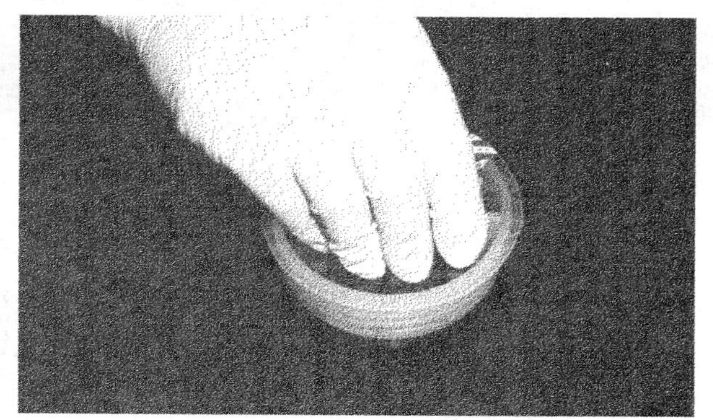

Surface Sampling Research Needed:

Validation of currently available and/or development of methods to establish protocols for optimal monitoring of biothreat scenarios.

Sample Analysis

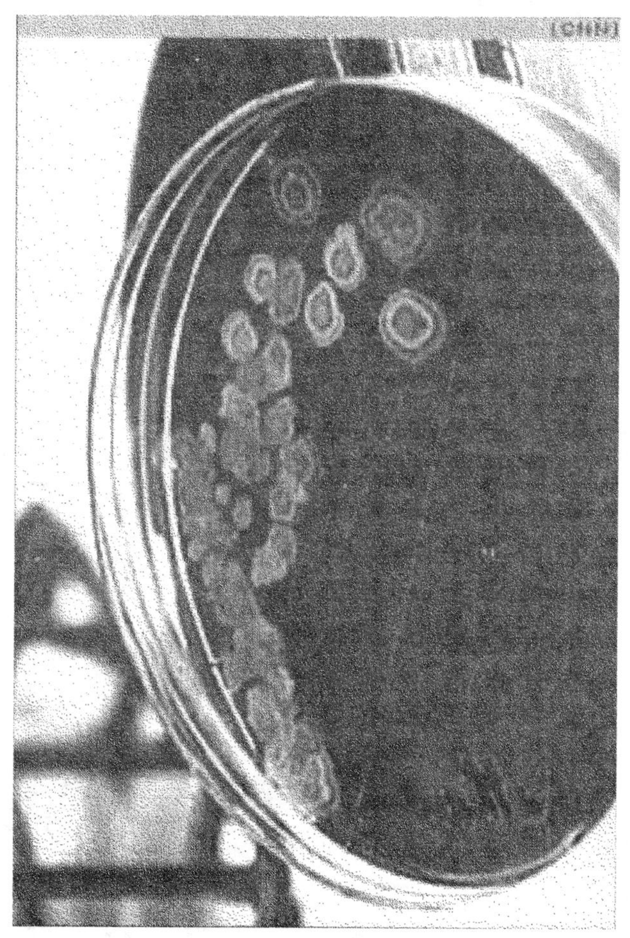

Molecular Biology Detection

- Rapid
- Sensitive
- Specific

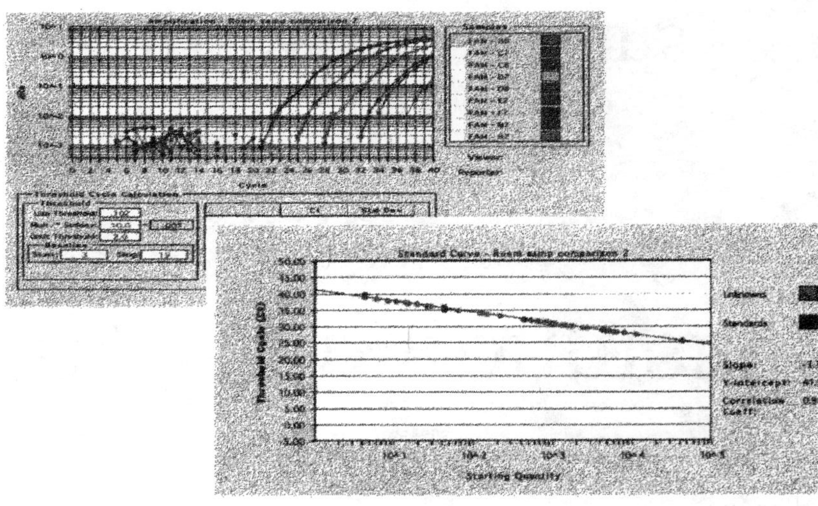

Interferences from Environmental Background

- Naturally-occurring organisms
- Dust, particulate
- Sampling materials

Information Needed:

- Background populations of biothreat agents and interferences outdoors and in enclosed public areas
  - Stadiums
  - Arenas
  - Convention centers
  - Public transportation facilities
  - Shopping centers

Increased University Research:

- Foundation studies already conducted
- Available facilities minimize start-up
- Less expensive
- Independent, no vested interest in any protocol

STETZENL@UNLV.NEVADA.EDU

Mr. SHAYS. It is pretty extraordinary that you would have been told in 1994 that once they settled, you didn't need to worry about the anthrax spores.

Dr. STETZENBACH. Pardon me. I didn't hear you.

Mr. SHAYS. It is pretty amazing to me that you were told, once anthrax spores had settled, they would not be a recurring problem. I mean, that's basically what you said, or did I——

Dr. STETZENBACH. That was the basic answer, yes, sir. And I said, "did you see my data," and he said, basically, "don't confuse me with the facts." It was unfortunate.

Mr. SHAYS. That was 4 years before—I mean 10 years earlier from now.

Dr. STETZENBACH. That was years earlier, yes, sir.

Mr. SHAYS. OK.

Chief Schwartz, welcome.

STATEMENT OF JAMES H. SCHWARTZ

Chief SCHWARTZ. Thank you, Mr. Chairman, members of the subcommittee.

In addition to my responsibilities as a fire chief in Arlington County, I am also a member of the Interagency Board for Equipment Standardization where I co-chair the Detection and Decontamination Subgroup. And I am also a member of the International Association of Fire Chiefs Committee on Terrorism and Homeland Security. These issues have great relevance for both of those groups.

I appreciate the opportunity to provide testimony on the issue of valid test methods for Bacillus anthracis today. This is a significant issue for Arlington County, which like most local governments, provide the public safety and public health response for our residents, visitors and businesses.

In Arlington, our services also protect the Pentagon and dozens of Federal agencies that reside in the over 60 percent of the county's available commercial office space, office space that I would observe is greater than what you will find in Baltimore, Seattle or San Francisco.

Arlington bears a significant responsibility for response to any incident that is perceived to have involved anthrax or other biological agents. I want to begin by complimenting the subcommittee on its charge to GAO regarding the assessment of postal facility testing and the validity of detection activities. This is a critical issue for local governments who, again, must manage the consequences of a local biological incident. But I would observe, it is not just postal facilities that we need to concentrate on.

Given our experience to date, I would also observe that there is no crisis that requires more accurate and timely public information than a public health crisis. Assuring the public, especially those who have been potentially exposed to a biological agent, is of the highest importance and makes reliable test results from a certified laboratory essential.

The decisions that result from testing, including the possible distribution of powerful antibiotics as prophylaxis, poses different but no less significant kinds of risk for the public.

I want to say that I agree with the recommendations of the GAO draft report which was provided to us. While the report describes significant hurdles to effective testing, it is imperative that methods of detecting anthrax and other biological hazards be developed so that appropriate decisions that are in the best interests of public health can be made in a timely way.

Special emphasis should also be put on environmental sampling methods. Detection methods have a considerable effect on the actions of local government. And as such, I want to take an opportunity to discuss briefly the incident at the Pentagon on March 14th, which I know you will be getting more testimony on in just a few moments. This incident was in many ways a model of inter-governmental cooperation.

Arlington County was notified of a possible test result at the Pentagon's remote delivery facility. Upon arrival at the facility, responders from Arlington learned that a swab taken from a filter 3 days earlier had tested positive for BA at a contract laboratory. Arlington committed its fire, police, public health and emergency management departments to support the Pentagon.

Because of our close working relationships with the Pentagon Force Protection Agency, we have a great deal of knowledge about their procedures. Numerous exercises over the last 7 years have helped to provide Arlington and the Pentagon Force Protection Agency with a better development system of planning and response.

In general, the response was good. The Pentagon Force Protection Agency notified Arlington as soon as they recognized a problem. And our first responders notified our Office of Emergency Management as soon as they arrived on the scene and assessed the situation.

Our Office of Emergency Management then made internal notifications and to other local governments in the region and the State. And I want to digress from my written testimony for just a moment here, because this morning, in hearing reports regarding the failure, the suggested failure of notification of the State in this particular incident, I believe that conclusion is largely flawed. Information went directly to the State from Arlington County's Office of Emergency Management as per protocols established by the Department of Homeland Security, soon after recognition that this was in fact an event, and our Office of Emergency Management took the next step by notifying the D.C. Emergency Management Agency to let them know what was going on as well.

As always, there are lessons to be learned from incidents such as this. While there are parts of the March 14th Pentagon response that could be improved upon, we are far beyond where we were 5 years ago. And I am confident that the after-action reports will bear that out. However, one of the salient points with this incident that the subcommittee focuses on today is valid detection methods.

Can we rely on the results we get from environmental sampling and subsequent laboratory analysis? Experts far smarter than I, I guess as you mentioned earlier, Mr. Chairman, smart science, will have to work out the answers to the challenges posed by the GAO report. But as a recipient of information derived from these practices, information on which critical public health and emergency management decisions can be made, I can say that the issue must be pursued.

In addition to the importance of valid testing methods of the postal facilities, I want to draw the subcommittee's attention to the importance of providing reliable screening technology for first responders.

The issue of testing for biological hazards has been a topic before the interagency board for over 3 years. First responders must have reliable biological detection capabilities. And I would ask that the subcommittee do everything it can to encourage the development of enhanced field-deployable technologies.

There are those in the Federal Government who would dismiss the need for this kind of capability in the hands of first responders. They insist that local first responders cannot be properly trained to use handheld assays or PCR technology and that responders should rely solely on the LRN to provide definitive results regarding the identification of suspicious substances. As my friend A.D. Vickery from Seattle Fire Department is fond of saying, this is the same argument we heard years ago when we were told that doctors only should be doing CPR.

The reality is that, on a frequent basis, first responders are called to investigate suspicious substances. This is especially true when the media is reporting a situation such as the one that occurred in Arlington and Fairfax several weeks ago. Simply relying on the LRN for test results is an ineffective way to provide timely advice and guidance to people who believe that they have been exposed to a biological agent.

First responders understand that there are more sophisticated field testing methods, that sophisticated field testing methods only yield presumptive results. We are not making clinical decisions with these methodologies but tactical decisions to manage public anxiety.

I will leave the remainder of my testimony in the written form and be happy to answer any questions that you may have.

[The prepared statement of Chief Schwartz follows:]

Anthrax Testing

Testimony

before the

**Subcommittee on National Security, Emerging Threats
and International Relations**

April 5, 2005

by

James H. Schwartz,

Fire Chief,

Arlington County, Virginia

Mr. Chairman and members of the committee, my name is James Schwartz and I am the Fire Chief for Arlington County Virginia. I am also a member of the Inter-Agency Board for Equipment Standardization and Interoperability where I serve as the co-chair of the Detection and Decontamination Sub-Group and I am a member of the International Association of Fire Chiefs Committee on Terrorism and Homeland Security.

I appreciate the opportunity to provide testimony on the issue of valid test methods for *Bacillus Anthracis*. This is a significant issue for Arlington County who, like most local governments, provide traditional public safety and public health first response for our residents, visitors and businesses. Unlike any other government, in Arlington our services also protect the Pentagon and dozens of federal agencies that reside in over 60 percent of the county's available commercial office space. Arlington bears significant responsibility for response to any incident that is perceived to involve anthrax or other biological hazards.

I want to begin by complimenting the subcommittee on its charge to GAO regarding the assessment of postal facility testing and the validity of detection activities. This is a critical issue for local governments who must manage the consequences of a biological incident, I would observe, not just at postal facilities. Given our experience to date, I would also observe that there is no crisis that requires more accurate and timely public information than a public health crisis. Assuring the public, especially those who may have been exposed to a biological agent, which is of the highest importance, makes reliable test results from a certified laboratory essential. The decisions that result from testing, including the possible distribution of powerful antibiotics as prophylaxis, poses different, but no less significant kinds of risk for the public.

I also want to say that I agree with the recommendations from the GAO draft report that was provided to us. While the report describes significant hurdles to effective testing, it is imperative that methods of detecting anthrax and other biological hazards be developed so that appropriate decisions that are in the best interest of public health can be made in a timely way. Special emphasis should be put on environmental sampling methods.

Detection methods have a considerable effect on the actions of local government. As such, I want to take this opportunity to discuss the incident at the Pentagon on Monday, March 14. This incident was in many ways a model of effective inter-governmental cooperation. Arlington County was notified of a possible positive test result at the Pentagon's remote delivery facility. Upon arrival at the delivery facility responders from Arlington learned that a swab taken from a filter three days earlier had tested positive for *Bacillus Anthracis* at a contract laboratory. Arlington committed its fire, police, public health and emergency management departments to support the Pentagon. Because of our close working relationships with the Pentagon Force Protection Agency (PFPA) Arlington personnel are aware of many of the Pentagon detection capabilities and procedures. Numerous exercises over the last seven years have helped to provide both Arlington and PFPA with a better developed system of planning and response.

In general the response was good. PFPA notified Arlington as soon they recognized a problem and our first responders notified our Office of Emergency Management as soon as they arrived on the scene and assessed the situation. OEM then made internal notifications and to other local governments in the region and the state.

As always there are lessons to be learned from incidents such as this. While there are parts of the March 14 Pentagon response that could be improved upon, we are far beyond where we were five years ago. I am confident that the after action reports currently being finalized will bear this out.

However, one of the salient points with this incident is the one the committee focuses on today; valid detection methods and adequate test protocols for anthrax. Can we rely on the results we get from environmental sampling and subsequent laboratory analysis? Experts far smarter than I will have to work out the answers to challenges posed by the GAO report, but as a recipient of information derived from these practices, information on which critical public health and emergency management decisions must be made, I can say that the issue must be pursued.

In addition to the importance of validating testing methods at postal facilities I want to draw the committee's attention to the importance of providing reliable screening technology for first responders. The issue of testing for biological hazards has been a topic before the Interagency Board for the last three years. First responders need reliable biological detection capabilities and I would ask that the committee do everything it can to encourage the development of enhanced field deployable technologies.

There are those in the federal government who dismiss the need for field detection of biological hazards. They insist that local first responders cannot be properly trained to use hand held assays and PCR technology and that first responders should rely solely on the Laboratory Response Network to provide definitive results regarding the identification of suspicious substances. As my friend A.D. Vickery from Seattle Fire Department is fond of saying, this is the same argument we heard years ago when we were told that only doctors should perform CPR.

The reality is that on a frequent basis first responders are called to investigate suspicious substances. This is especially true when the media is reporting a situation such as the one Arlington and Fairfax experienced a few weeks ago. It seems that attention to these types of incidents heightens anxieties and adds confusion. First responders must manage this public anxiety and the effective use of field detection is a way to ensure that this can be accomplished. Simply relying on the LRN for test results is an ineffective way of providing timely advice and guidance to people who believe that they have been exposed to a biological agent. First responders understand very well that the most sophisticated field testing methods yield only presumptive results and that confirmatory tests from a certified laboratory are required to make more definitive public health decisions. Nonetheless, it is incomprehensible that some would have responders telling dozens or hundreds of nervous and worried people that the earliest information is 24-hours away.

In Arlington we have gone to great lengths to ensure that our field detection capabilities are used to make tactical, not clinical decisions. We do this by beginning each response with a threat assessment. This assessment is conducted with our local police department and/or the FBI. If it is determined that a legitimate threat is present, appropriate first steps can be taken to inform and protect the public. Our procedures were developed jointly with fire, police, emergency management and public health at the table and we constantly review those procedures to ensure they are as up to date as possible.

The fact is that first responders need field detection capabilities to make tactical decisions; no first responder I know of is advocating the use of field detection for clinical decision making. This is the role of public health authorities and is where the LRN is so valuable. Several years ago when communities were experiencing the first "white powder" incidents, there were few laboratories that were recognized as capable of doing effective confirmatory tests. First responders were much more on there own, flying in the dark with little to no technical back-up. While the network has become a valuable national asset it should not be seen as a universal remedy.

Arlington, along with our partners in the region, has been on the forefront of terrorism preparedness. In 1997 we, along with our partners in the region, established the nation's first civilian terrorism response team, known then as the Metropolitan Medical Strike Team. Staffed with emergency medical, hazmat, and law enforcement personnel from jurisdictions around the national capital region, the team, now known as the National Medical Response Team, provides a unique response capability that includes mass casualty decontamination and its own cache of pharmaceuticals.

Following the creation of this response team, it became apparent that a more systematic approach was necessary, one that required an integration of planning and response and that included public health and hospitals. This integration does not come about only through the use of unified incident management once an incident is recognized. It must start with integrated planning that is done across professional disciplines. From that understanding the Metropolitan Medical Response System was born. MMRS now exists in 122 communities across the country.

This systematic approach integrates the planning and response of first responders (fire, EMS, hazmat and law enforcement), including public health, emergency management and hospitals and medical care facilities to work together to develop the capability to reduce the human health consequences which result from terrorist acts. It also requires concurrent integration with neighboring jurisdictions and State and Federal agencies.

It is important to underscore the fact that incidents such as those we experienced in October of 2001, again in November of 2003 and then again a few weeks ago at the Pentagon and in Fairfax County, require a public safety and public health response that is integrated.

MMRS is one of the best approaches ever devised for regional planning and response to a large scale incident. We think MMRS should be considered as a national model for how local governments should plan and organize for a large scale incident where mass casualties are involved, as well as to address the additional hazards that an integrated approach to planning affords.

Unfortunately, the Administration did not include MMRS in its fiscal 2006 budget submittal. As you deliberate today and in the near term about improving the nation's preparedness I urge you to support additional funding for MMRS. It is critical to our ability to protect our citizens as well as DOD and other federal employees in this region—so we need your leadership and guidance in order to have certainty that our efforts may proceed.

I hope that my comments today are helpful and I appreciate your consideration of them. I am confident that they reflect some of the problems faced by first responders not just in Arlington, but across the country. I look forward to answering any questions you might have.

Mr. SHAYS. Thank you very, very much.

Chief Neuhard.

STATEMENT OF MICHAEL P. NEUHARD

Chief NEUHARD. Thank you, Mr. Chairman. I will note that I have provided some lengthy testimony in writing, and I will summarize that very quickly here for you.

Mr. SHAYS. Thank you very much.

Chief NEUHARD. Mr. Chairman, distinguished members of the subcommittee. I am Michael Neuhard, and I am the fire chief of the Fairfax County Fire and Rescue Department, which is located in the northern Virginia area of the National Capital Region. We appreciate this opportunity to provide you with a local perspective on anthrax detection and the problems associated with first responder activities during potential anthrax incidents.

During the last 4 years, Fairfax County and other regional agencies have had the unfortunate occasion to respond to over 1,000 potential anthrax incidents. As you are aware, we recently responded to a detection device activation at a Department of Defense facility located in Fairfax County, which occurred simultaneously with a potential anthrax incident at the Pentagon, Arlington County, VA.

Our experience at these incidents shows that, at the most fundamental level, the question of determining if we are dealing with a biological agent in an accurate and timely manner remains elusive. We believe there are four areas relevant to this hearing in the anthrax detection chain which presents significant challenges during the first 72 hours of an incident.

First is the current state of fixed detection systems being operated in local jurisdictions at government mail-handling facilities. Fixed mail-handling facilities are using different detection technologies with varying degrees of reliability. In many instances, the instance and type of device is not known to nor coordinated with local officials. Furthermore, these facilities may not even have technical support available for these detectors after normal business hours.

On a positive note, a postal facility in Fairfax County has worked very diligently with officials to develop joint protocols for response to an activation of their biological detection system. Conversely, when the 911 call was received for the DOD facility on Leesburg Pike, first responders were not even aware that a detection device was located within the facility.

The second issue is the lack of reliable field screening capabilities for first responders, as was noted by Chief Schwartz. None of the field test devices on the market today are endorsed by scientists or laboratories as being reliable, accurate and consistent. This prevents the first responders from having appropriate, technical information to support initial decisions in the field, and all of us know the consequences of that.

The third issue is obtaining the laboratory results and ensuring that they are available for decisionmakers during an incident. Once field samples have been transported to a laboratory, local and State officials are not fully aware of nor included in the process. Many times and most of the time, our experience has been these have gone to Federal laboratories.

During the recent simultaneous events, it was difficult to determine which location or sample, testing procedures or time lines the subject matter experts were referring to as they attempted to make decisions and articulate this to local and State representatives. This problem leads to local and State responders making decisions based on limited and sometimes unreliable information.

Finally, the lack of confidence in the ability of the laboratories to produce timely, accurate and reliable analysis is troubling. Since emergency responders have limited ability to identify a potential biological agent in the field, they rely heavily on the testing laboratories for accurate and timely information.

It is unconscionable that a laboratory can provide positive screening and culture test results for a biological agent that was not present. At a minimum, laboratories utilized for routine and incident specific samples should be certified in part of the laboratory response network. Additionally, initial test results should be available to decisionmakers within 4 to 6 hours as opposed to the 12 to 15 hours indicated during recent events.

It is imperative that Federal, State and local authorities partner in efforts to improve detection, screening and analysis of potential anthrax contamination. The Federal Government can help by insuring, first, that all stakeholders are at the table as we further refine these capabilities, the local, State and Federal levels together. Second, provide ample funding to continue research that enables reliable, consistent and timely detection, field screening and lab analysis.

Third, require Federal agencies operating fixed detection systems in localities to coordinate with local first responders and public health officials. And, finally, ensure that Federal agencies ensure similar protocols across Federal agency lines in the detection and response to potential anthrax incidents.

While the Federal Government must continue to provide leadership in the anthrax response arena, it must remember that when an incident strikes, it is the localities that would be impacted and challenged with the appropriate response. We must recognize this and accept this, and we must do everything possible to provide appropriate technical capabilities so we can answer as quickly and confidently as possible the question, do we have anthrax?

Thank you.

[The prepared statement of Chief Neuhard follows:]

Anthrax Detection: A Local Perspective

Testimony by Chief Michael P. Neuhard
Fairfax County Fire and Rescue Department

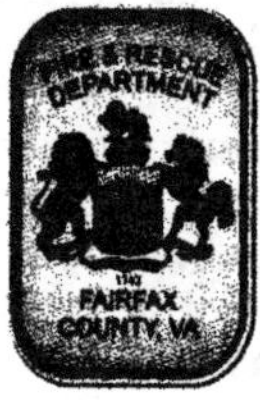

Before the House Government Reform Subcommittee on National Security, Emergency Threats, and International Relations

Tuesday, April 5, 2005

Anthrax Detection: A Local Perspective

Testimony by Chief Michael P. Neuhard
Fairfax County Fire and Rescue Department
before the House Government Reform Subcommittee on National Security,
Emerging Threats, and International Relations

Tuesday, April 5, 2005

Introduction

Chairman Shays, distinguished members of the Subcommittee, my name is Michael P. Neuhard, and I am the Fire Chief for the Fairfax County Fire and Rescue Department located in the Northern Virginia area of the National Capital Region. Thank you for the opportunity to provide you with a local perspective on anthrax detection and the problems associated with first responder activities during potential anthrax emergencies.

The Fairfax County Fire and Rescue Department serves over one million residents, as well as workers in local businesses and industry, and transient visitors who pass through our jurisdiction on one of the interstate highways that traverse our County. We provide emergency service through a network of 35 strategically placed fire stations and a staff of over 1800 dedicated men and women. Our stations are staffed 24 hours a day, 7 days a week, 365 days a year. We are an all-hazard fire department, providing fire suppression services, basic life support (BLS) and advanced life support (ALS) emergency medical services, and technical specialties to include specialized rescue and cave-in capabilities, hazardous materials response and mitigation and marine operations. The Department also provides fire and hazardous materials preventative services through its Fire Marshal's Office. We respond to approximately 90,000 calls for service a year and our call volume continues to grow.

I provide you with this information as background for a sense of the depth and scope of the services provided in a large urban area that has benefited from the efforts of regional cooperation and coordination. We continue to work toward achieving cooperation and coordination among our diverse jurisdictions in Northern Virginia and the Metropolitan Washington region. In addition, because of our proximity to Washington, DC, and the potential targets this area presents, we have been fortunate enough to receive federal funding support toward our goals of planning, preparedness, response, and mitigation activities for all types of emergencies, but especially for expanding WMD response capabilities.

Background

During the last four years, Fairfax County, in conjunction with the region, has had the unfortunate occasion to respond to thousands of potential anthrax incidents. These have included letters sent through the mail, threats, and fixed detection system alerts that have resulted in death, illness, public hysteria, and disruption to critical infrastructure. Recently, a detection device activated at a Department of Defense (DOD) facility located at 5111 Leesburg Pike, which occurred simultaneously with a potential anthrax incident at the Pentagon in Arlington County, Virginia. These experiences, along with an increase in training, development of operational procedures, and use of technology have provided us an opportunity to face and understand the challenges, issues, and problems associated with the response to potential anthrax incidents. We have made significant strides since the fall of 2001; however, in some areas we still have considerable room for improvement. Efforts toward coordination and cooperation during an incident continue to be strengthened through federal programs and local initiatives. Interoperability of communications is being addressed, incident management principles consistent with the National Incident Management System (NIMS) are being implemented, notification methods and techniques are being designed, implemented, and improved upon. Likewise, considerable effort has been put into field detection, screening, and analysis for potential biological agents. While there is much room to improve in all of these areas, our recent experience shows that at the most fundamental level, the question of determining if we are dealing with a biological agent in an accurate and timely manner remains elusive. Current anthrax detection, field screening, and lab analysis does not provide local emergency responders, public health officials, or law enforcement with timely, accurate, and reliable information upon which to base decisions about public health and safety.

Anthrax Detection Issues

Based on our experience in Fairfax County we believe there are four areas in the anthrax detection chain which present significant challenges during the first 72-hours of an incident. These issues reside in the following areas:

First, is the current state of fixed detection systems being operated in local jurisdictions at government mail handling facilities. Fixed mail handling facilities are using different detection technologies with varying degrees of reliability. These devices use different screening methods, and widely different protocols. In many instances, the placement of these devices is not coordinated with local officials and in some cases, the existence of the machines may not be known. Additionally, the type of device being utilized and again protocols in use may not be known to local responders. Furthermore, these facilities may not even have information or technical support available for these detectors after normal business hours, even during an emergency incident. For example, there is a postal facility in Fairfax County that has worked very diligently with officials to develop joint protocols for response to an activation of their biological detection system (BDS.) This includes identifying roles and responsibilities of each entity during the initial response. Conversely, when the 911 call was received for the the DOD facility on Leesburg Pike, first responders were not even aware that a detection device was located within the facility, responders were not aware that old technology (particle counter) was being used as the detection device. Furthermore, there were no joint or collaborative protocols in place for this facility, a stark contrast from our postal facility agreement.

The second issue is the lack of reliable field screening capabilities for first responders. Currently first responders of any type, i.e., fire and rescue, public heath, and law enforcement, have only limited methods available to them to conduct field screening of anthrax or other biological agents. None of the field test devices on the market are endorsed by scientists or laboratories as being reliable, accurate, and consistent. This prevents the first responders from having appropriate technical information to support decisions in the field.

The third issue is obtaining the laboratory results of samples and ensuring that they are available for decision makers during an incident. Once field samples have been taken and transported to a laboratory, which in many instances is a federal facility, local and state officials are not fully aware of, nor included in the process. This includes not knowing all of the participating agencies, i.e., United States Army Medical Research Institute for Infectious Diseases (USAMRIID) Centers for Disease Control and Prevention (CDC), DOD, etc., the status of the samples, the time-line for definitive results, nor the actual process for obtaining the results so they can be utilized for critical decision making. During the recent events, it is questionable whether the federal decision makers understood where in the process the samples were as they attempted to make decisions and articulate this to the local/state representatives. It was difficult with two simultaneous events to determine which of the locations samples, testing procedures, and time-lines the subject matter experts were referring to. This problem leads to local/state responders making decisions based on no information, inadequate information, and sometimes unreliable information. This exacerbates the stress on the potential victims and complicates the decisions to provide prophylaxis medications, reoccupy and open buildings, and convey the appropriate message to the public.

And finally, the lack of confidence in the ability of laboratories to produce timely, accurate, and reliable analysis is troubling. Since emergency responders have limited ability to identify a potential biological agent in the field, they rely heavily on the testing laboratories for accurate and timely information. It is unconscionable that a laboratory could provide positive polymerase chain reaction (PCR) and culture test results for a biological agent that was not present. These tainted findings produced a tremendous hardship on the occupants of 5111 Leesburg Pike, increased public concern, had an adverse impact on the building/infrastructure, and consumed public safety resources unnecessarily. At a minimum, it is expected that laboratories utilized for routine and incident-specific samples should be certified, and part of the laboratory response network. Anything less is unacceptable. Additionally, initial results, i.e., PCR for emergency incidents, should be available to decision makers within 4 to 6 hours as opposed to the 12-15 hours indicated during the recent events.

Conclusion

We have come along way since the fall of 2001 with our capabilities to detect, respond to, and mitigate potential anthrax threats. But as discussed today, there is still much work to be done. It is imperative that the federal, state, and local authorities partner in these efforts to improve detection, screening, sampling, and analysis of potential anthrax contamination. The federal government can help by ensuring (1) all the stakeholders are at the table as we further refine capabilities; (2) provide ample funding to continue research that ensures reliable, consistent, and timely detection, field screening, sampling, transportation, and lab analysis; (3) require federal agencies operating detection systems in localities to coordinate with local first responders and

- 4 -

public health officials; and (4) ensure that federal agencies employ similar protocols across federal agency lines in the detection of a response to potential anthrax incidents (unified federal approach).

While the federal government must continue to provide leadership in the anthrax response arena, it must remember that when an incident strikes, it is the localities, the local citizens, the local government, the local response agencies, and local health agencies that will be impacted and challenged with the appropriate response. We must recognize this, we must accept this, and we must do everything possible to provide appropriate detection, screening, and analysis so we can answer as quickly and as confidently as possible the question, <u>do we have anthrax here</u>? Thank you very much.

Mr. SHAYS. Thank you, Chief Neuhard.

Mr. Schaenman. Am I pronouncing your name correctly?

STATEMENT OF PHILIP SCHAENMAN

Mr. SCHAENMAN. Schaenman, yes. Thank you again and the members of the subcommittee for inviting me to this important hearing. I will give you a quick verbal summary of the written testimony. I am Philip Schaenman, president of the Tridata Division of System Planning Corp.

We have been providing analytical services dealing with public safety for about 35 years. We have done over 50 after-action reports for major public safety incidents. And we have evaluated public safety services at about 150 communities and 40 Navy installations.

About 2 weeks ago, State and local officials in Virginia, Maryland and D.C. voiced concerns about the information flow, as well as the science—as you have been talking about—during the suspected anthrax incidents. They wanted a rapid after-action review of the State and local actions and information flow by an expert third party in parallel with the Federal studies that were being done of the time lines and what happened. And I got tagged with being the project manager. Here is a brief summary of the findings, focusing on the information flow rather than the science.

Overall, the National Capital Region did much better than it would have been 5 years ago. Arlington and Fairfax County did extremely well in responding to the incidents, in communicating with each other and in sending information to the region, as Chief Schwartz said.

The Commonwealth of Virginia was prepared to assist its counties. The State of Maryland was prepared and kept informed. D.C. government was prepared and played a direct role at the V Street facility. So the overall picture was good, but there were many communication problems identified. Most of them stemmed from the root cause of not having clear information about the status and findings of the anthrax tests.

But in a sense, that's the homeland security version of the fog of war. You need to be able to deal with the uncertainty in these types of incidents.

For one thing, there needs to be better protocols on who has responsibilities for keeping the region informed, beyond the jurisdictions directly involved. Should a county pass information to the National Capital Region or to the Department of Homeland Security for dissemination into the rest of the region.

Mr. SHAYS. You have to move your mic back just a speck. Please just slide it back.

Mr. SCHAENMAN. Sorry.

Mr. SHAYS. No need to apologize. You are doing great.

Mr. SCHAENMAN. So how should the information flow? Should it go from the State through the region, or should it go to DHS and then through the region? Should it go from office of emergency management to office of emergency management that are the hubs and in through the spokes, or should it be broadcast to all agencies simultaneously? Should it go public health to public health and fire to fire?

Well the problem in these incidents, I went through all these channels. And it led to uncertainty as to what was the latest and most authoritative information at any given time, in part because the tests weren't clearly defined and time stamped as the information flowed across agencies.

There were times when 80 people were on a conference call being updated without knowing what the source of the information was, whether that was the most recent information and whether they could ask questions or not, so they had little idea of the validity of the information at times.

Another issue that needs guidance from the State and local chief executives is when they want to be informed about incidents that are not yet confirmed. There was hesitancy about passing information up the line, but generally good judgment.

But people are concerned about the boy who cries wolf syndrome on the one hand and, on the other hand, keeping political leadership informed before they hear about it from CNN. A balance needs to be struck.

There is also a need to more forthrightly inform the public on what is going on even in the face of uncertainty. It's probably better to say we have conflicting test information and trying to resolve it than delaying press releases all together, and that happened.

There needs to be greater care in the use of English language and acronyms in emergency communications. We have been working the problem of interoperability of the hardware of communications, but there's an interoperability problem on the human side as well. For example, there was communication that it had set off an automatic alarm at Skyline Towers when it was in fact a person giving an alarm. And there's a big difference. There was a misunderstanding about whether a test was for the presence of anthrax spores or for the viability of anthrax spores, and that's a difference.

DOD, several State and local agencies felt that DOD needed to better coordinate medical treatment decisions with their public health agencies, in this case Pentagon with Arlington County, but elsewhere in the Nation as well. And it affects people in the local jurisdiction.

So those are just some of the key findings. We are going to have detailed time lines and findings from the point of view of all the major State and local government participants in a report that's forthcoming. I would be glad to answer questions.

[The prepared statement of Mr. Schaenman follows:]

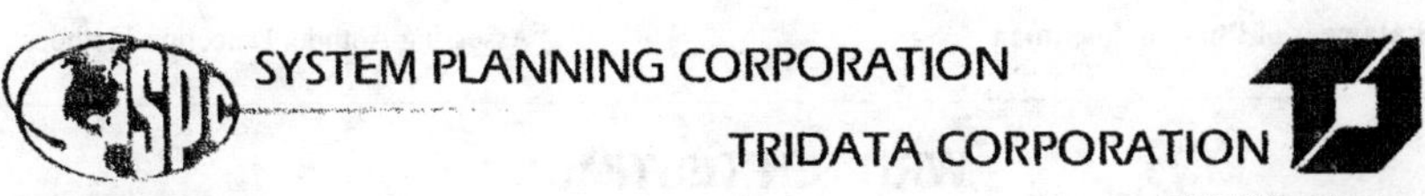

SYSTEM PLANNING CORPORATION

TRIDATA CORPORATION

1000 Wilson Boulevard
Arlington, Virginia 22209
(703) 351-8200
Fax: (703) 351-8311
http://www.sysplan.com

1000 Wilson Boulevard
Arlington, Virginia 22209
(703) 351-8300
Fax: (703) 351-8383
http://www.tridatacorp.com

STATEMENT OF

Philip Schaenman, President
TriData, a Division of
System Planning Corporation
Arlington, Virginia

BEFORE THE

Subcommittee on National Security, Emerging
Threats, and International Relations
COMMITTEE ON GOVERNMENT REFORM
U.S. House of Representatives

ON

"Assessing Anthrax Detection Methods"

April 5, 2005

WRITTEN TESTIMONY

Thank you, Mr. Chairman and members of the subcommittee, for inviting me to participate in this important hearing.

I am Philip Schaenman, president of the TriData division of System Planning Corporation (SPC). I was Associate Administrator of the U.S. Fire Administration in its early days and am an engineer by training.

Corporate Background

SPC has been providing emergency and analytical services to governments at all levels for over 35 years. We have undertaken over 50 after-action reports for FEMA and other agencies, and have evaluated public safety services in over 150 communities and 40 U.S. Navy installations. SPC is one of the few companies that has in-depth experience in both national-level homeland security issues and public safety in state and local governments.

We work directly with local, state, and federal agencies and their personnel in the interdiction, response, and consequence management areas. SPC understands the different perspectives and mission assignments of each and effectively communicates with all.

SPC is composed of two major divisions, the System Technology Division, which, among other things, develops instrumentation radar and flight termination systems and the National Intelligence, Security, and Response (NISR) division, of which TriData is a component.

The NISR division provides a broad range of homeland security services including data collection and analysis; performance measurement and management; local public safety evaluations; and the activity that brings me here today, after-action reviews and analysis of major incidents and exercises.

The Incidents

Key local and state officials in Virginia, Maryland, and the District of Columbia voiced concerns about the timeliness and accuracy of the information flow during the suspected anthrax incidents of March 11–15, 2005. They decided to charter a rapid after-action review of local and state actions by an objective third party, in parallel with a planned Department of Homeland Security (DHS) study of federal agency actions and timelines. SPC was selected on March 17 to undertake the urgent one-week study. The task was assigned to our TriData division and I served as project manager.

The incidents tested the readiness of emergency communications and response systems in National Capital Region (NCR) local governments and two states for a biological attack, and the approaches for disseminating information among local, state, and federal agencies and to the public.

The basic objectives of this study were to determine when and how various entities of state and local government learned about the incidents and how information then flowed between federal, state, and local levels. The goals were to determine how well the information exchange worked and how it could be improved in the future.

Key Findings

The following is a summary of the key findings of our study. A parallel DHS study considered federal agency actions and information flow.

Positives

1. Arlington County and Fairfax County governments are battle-hardened in homeland security and performed extremely well both on the ground and in terms of information flow.

2. Overall, the entire emergency management complex at the state and local levels acted professionally. There was generally good state and local interagency cooperation and communication. The emergency responses were good and the information flow much better than would have been the case even 5 years ago. Many aspects of communications could improve, but most of the essentials were in place.

3. The two principal counties involved (Arlington and Fairfax) did an outstanding job of communicating within themselves, and with each other.

4. The State agencies in Virginia and Maryland were mobilized and ready to support the local governments. These jurisdictions used many resources to keep informed and be supportive as needed.

5. The State of Maryland and District of Columbia mobilized quickly and adequately monitored the developing situation. They used good judgment in how far to go in the light of uncertainty and the potential impacts of the incident.

Concerns and Issues to Be Resolved

While the big picture was good, there were many communication issues.

1. *Was it a real attack?* – The major information flow and operational problems centered on the lack of clarity as to whether there was anthrax present or not, what tests had been performed, what the results were, and what they meant. The problem was compounded by the more subtle problem of not adequately communicating the level of uncertainty about the status of the anthrax tests.

2. *Does any agency have the latest information?* The state and local governments were not sure if they were getting the latest and best information from the Department of Defense (DoD), or whether DoD itself was having problems obtaining clear test information, or both.

3. *How should information flow beyond the jurisdiction of origin?* – When a local government has an incident, who should they inform external to themselves and how should they pass on the information? Local to state to NCR? Local to NCR to state to all locals? Should flow go from office of emergency management to office of emergency management and then to each network coordinated by each OEM? Or should information flow by discipline, e.g., health department to health department, police to police, fire to fire, etc.? Essentially all of the above paths were used in just a two-day period. Each discipline has its own protocols for alerts and updates. State agencies have formed policies that local governments are expected to follow. A region-wide protocol needs to be established to ensure timely information flow and reduce redundancy. State and local laws regarding emergency information need to be considered in the protocols. There are differences of opinion state to state and among the counties on what should be the prime path of communication and alerting. That needs to be resolved.

4. *Over-Communicating?* – In part, there was a problem of over-communicating (too many people getting information from too many sources) without being sure one had the latest information in a continually changing biological testing situation. The large numbers of people and agencies involved in sending and receiving information, especially multiple, large scale conference calls, made it difficult at times for the key actors to exchange information on the test findings, and to have time to act on it.

5. ***Early DHS Involvement*** – The state and local governments felt that the DHS needs to be involved earlier in such incidents, and that they all should have been informed by the DoD Pentagon earlier. According to some state and local agencies, the DHS/NCR should have been the prime agency to spread the word earlier to the region to ensure credibility and clarify information flow. (Others felt the information should be distributed by the state.)

6. ***Boy Who Cried Wolf Versus Giving Early Warning*** – Another issue to resolve is the balance between notifying stakeholders about a potential but unconfirmed threat too soon, causing undue concern and wasted actions , versus getting all relevant parties informed as soon as possible in case the threat turns out to be real. Early notice helps in making preparations and avoiding political embarrassment. But if false alarms occur too often, it can be detrimental. There needs to be discussions and decisions at the chief executive level (governors, mayors, county chief administrators) as to when they should be alerted and how far to go in setting up emergency operations centers and taking other steps for various levels of information. Some steps in information flow plans depend on the jurisdiction of origin deciding on whether it is a "significant" incident, but "significant" is not defined, even qualitatively, and it needs to be. In this incident, good judgment was generally exercised by state and local governments on passing along information, but with much uncertainty as to whether the right thing was being done (setting up emergency operations centers, informing chief executives, putting out press releases, etc.).

7. ***Public Health Decision-Making*** – Public health leaders must have early involvement in notification and decisionmaking on medical issues. When antibiotic prophylaxis decisions are made, local public health agencies must be able to assess the threat, perform epidemiological assessment, ready patient assessment and care personnel, tools, and facilities, and be able to offer other organizations access to resources. Fairfax, Arlington, and Commonwealth health officials felt that the public health coordination with DoD health officials was not adequate, especially regarding the decision to use prophylactic drugs on those who might have been exposed, before the problem was confirmed. Localities want to be involved in medical decisions affecting their constituents.

8. ***Large-Scale Conference Calls Need To Have More Structure and Order*** – Teleconferences should be conducted in an orderly and meaningful manner. Conference sponsors should determine who needs to participate and exclude others. The information needs to be more structured, and terminology used carefully, especially on the tests that were undertaken and their results. The 80-person conference calls were considered disorderly by almost everyone we interviewed. One individual, a "net control," needs to manage the call, make announcements, and then poll specific agencies. Call participants should not be allowed to speak free-lance; the participating agencies can assign one spokesperson, and they can be polled for questions by the moderator. There also is telephone technology to allow moderators to identify who wants to ask a question.

9. ***Timing of Public Information Releases*** – Coordination, timeliness, and content of public information release were not a total success here. Public information officials were concerned about releasing information about a muddy picture. It was often unclear as to what was fact, but that could have been explained to the public. Reliable internet sources for the media and public were not adequately established. The Joint Information Center might have been set up earlier and maintained longer. At least general information on the uncertainty of the situation could have been released earlier, along with general information on anthrax. One can tell the public what one knows at an earlier point in time and that the situation may change.

10. ***Sources of Regional Information*** – Federal agencies should use the appropriate, federally promulgated alerting systems for disasters. Some local and state officials felt that the DoD Pentagon should have notified the Homeland Security Operating Center (HSOC) in a more timely manner. The HSOC would quickly gather preliminary information and alert the appropriate state and local authorities. Others felt that DoD should notify the nearby jurisdictions and the state directly. The alert should consist of an incident summary, threats, and an initial recommendation for action. Getting an alert from a pre-arranged route makes it clearer to state and local officials that it is real and not a rumor.

11. ***Time to Validate Information*** – Information accuracy is crucial to state and local governments charged with providing emergency responses. In this instance, it took several days for emergency management leaders to get

enough information to determine the validity of the threat and the alerting mechanisms that were used (detection alarms, collected samples, human interaction, observations, etc.).

12. ***Consistency with NIMS*** – The federal government should assure that incident operations are in line with the National Incident Management System (NIMS).

13. ***Identifying Employees at Risk*** – Federal agencies must assure that notification procedures are in place so that private or contracted agencies can identify their employees at risk.

Timelines for key communications and more details on issues concerning information flow are available in the forthcoming report, "Anthrax Incidents in the National Capital Region, State and Local Government After-Action Review," dated March 29, 2005, prepared by System Planning Corporation for the Commonwealth of Virginia, District of Columbia, and State of Maryland. The report includes timelines and viewpoints from all the major participating state and local governments, and a number of recommendations.

Thank you again Mr. Chairman for inviting me to participate in this important hearing. I would be pleased to discuss the results of our review with you and your colleagues and respond to any questions.

Mr. SHAYS. Thank you.

Mr. Jester.

STATEMENT OF JOHN N. JESTER

Mr. JESTER. Mr. Chairman, members of the subcommittee, thank you.

My name is John Jester. I am the Director of the Pentagon Force Protection Agency. Thank you for inviting me to discuss the emergency response activities to the suspected anthrax contamination at the Pentagon's Defense Post Office and at a mail office in Skyline Tower 5.

In addition to a brief summary of events, I also plan on sharing with the subcommittee lessons learned and actions taken since the event. Overall, I want to assure the subcommittee that the Pentagon is an equal partner with the Federal, State and local entities in protecting the health and safety of our employees and the surrounding communities.

To briefly summarize the recent events, on Thursday, March 10th, Vistronix, a U.S. Army contractor, screened mail entering the Defense Post Office over down-draft tables. Swab samples taken from the filters under the tables were collected and sent to the Commonwealth Biotechnology Inc. Laboratory, hereafter referred to as CBI Lab. Standard procedures call for the contractor to hold the mail in quarantine mail for 3 days until the lab reports negative results.

At 4 p.m. on Friday, March 11, representatives from the CBI Lab informed the Vistronix site supervisor that the initial test result of Thursday's mail sample would be delayed due to a preliminary positive test result.

The Vistronix supervisor did not inform DOD of this preliminary test result. Over the weekend, CBI performed a confirmation test on the sample. On Monday morning, March 14, 6:15 a.m., Vistronix released Thursday's mail to the Defense Post Office for distribution. Three hours later, the CBI Lab informed the Vistronix supervisor that the test results from one of the samples from Friday's mail resulted in a positive response for anthrax.

The Defense Post Office was notified of the positive test results, immediately shut down their facility and immediately notified the Pentagon Force Protection Agency. In the 2 hours that followed, we established a secure perimeter around the remote delivery facility, notified Arlington County and set up an instant command post integrating local and Federal emergency response efforts; 236 employees from the remote delivery facility were evacuated to a nearby vacant building until they could be briefed, tested and issued precautionary treatment, and offered counseling services.

We coordinated with other Pentagon distribution offices to identify all possible recipients of the morning mail and deployed our HAZMAT teams to the sites for additional swab sample tests. Between 10 a.m. and 1 p.m., Pentagon Force Protection Agency notified State and local, Federal emergency response agencies of the potential biohazard incident through the Washington Area Warning System.

By 1 p.m., the Centers for Disease Control and Prevention, the Homeland Security Operation Center and the Office of the U.S.

Postmaster General were all notified. The Arlington County Fire Department arrived at the Pentagon 11:04 a.m., and the FBI was on the scene by 1 p.m.

Over the next 3 days, Pentagon officials coordinated with local, State and Federal officials, health and law enforcement officials. At approximately 2 p.m., we were notified that a bio alarm was set up in a mail distribution office in Skyline 5. It was later determined that the room in question did not have a biosensor or bioalarm.

The device was a biological air filtration hood, and the alarm was simply a red light indicating air flow restriction. All subsequent tests returned negative, and the Skyline Complex and the Remote Delivery Facility reopened on Thursday, March 17th. By Thursday, March 17th, the DiLorenzo Clinic in the Pentagon tested more than 800 people through nasal swabs and provided 3 days of antibiotics.

As in any emergency, there were actions that went very well and procedures that need to be improved. Our initial after-action assessments identified some positive aspects of the collective Pentagon response to this incident. The remote delivery facility as designed kept potentially harmful substances isolated from the large Pentagon population.

We immediately identified and screened potentially contaminated employees. Within 3 hours, our organic HAZMAT team conducted 130 tests of the mail room and other suspected areas.

Not everything transpired as it should have. It took too long for the original contractor lab mail results to be processed, and the contractor staff failed to follow mail release protocols. Additionally, there was no way to confirm that all State, local and Federal agencies heard the Washington Area Warning System message. The event illustrated that incidents at high-profile symbolic Federal facilities become breaking news stories and are quickly perceived as national events.

We have already taken major steps to address these issues. Since the suspected anthrax incident, Pentagon Force Protection Agency has assumed responsibility for the oversight of the mail screening process and testing the samples from filters at our Pentagon laboratory. The onsite lab provides 24-hour response for positive initial screening of multiple threat agents.

The Pentagon Force Protection Agency will ensure that mail is properly quarantined until the Pentagon lab returns negative sample test results. Revised notifications, both interagency and external, are in place for future chem-bioevents. Our procedures for using the Washington Area Warning System now include a preamble with an emergency message stating the who, what, where and when of the event. We will ensure that a response is received from an appropriate agency such as DHS, FBI and local counties. In 30 to 45 seconds, the emergency message will be repeated.

A thorough review and the assessment of the ability to response to and management of the incidents is being conducted. DOD will receive a draft after-action report in 21 days and a final report within 45 days. The Pentagon is fortunate to have an excellent working relationship with Arlington and Fairfax Counties' police and fire departments. These working relationships were tested and proven on September 11th and continue to improve as we participate in annual exercises.

Mr. Chairman, this concludes my prepared remarks. Thank you for the opportunity to speak, and I will be happy to answer any questions.

[The prepared statement of Mr. Jester follows:]

Summary and Actions Taken Since March 14, 2005 Anthrax Incident
Before the Subcommittee on National Security, Emerging Threats, and International Relations

Statement of John N. Jester, Director
Pentagon Force Protection Agency

Mr. Chairman and Members of the Subcommittee:

Thank you for inviting me to discuss the emergency response activities to the suspected anthrax contamination at the Pentagon's Defense Post Office (DPO) and at a mail office in Skyline Tower 5. In addition to a brief summary of events, I also plan on sharing with the Committee lessons learned and actions taken since the event. Overall, I want to reassure the Committee that the Pentagon is an equal partner with federal, state and local entities in protecting the health and safety of our employees and the surrounding communities. As a way of introduction, I am John N. Jester, Director of the Pentagon Force Protection Agency. We are responsible for the protection of the people, facilities, and infrastructure on the Pentagon Reservation. We perform a mission very similar to the U.S. Capitol Police.

SUMMARY

To briefly summarize the recent events; on Thursday, March 10, Vistronix, a U.S. Army contractor, screened mail entering the Defense Post Office over down-draft tables. Swab samples off the filters under the tables were collected and sent to the Commonwealth Biotechnology Incorporated Laboratory, hereafter, referred to as the CBI Lab. Standard procedures call for the contractor to hold the mail in quarantine for three days until the lab reports negative results.

At 4:00pm on Friday, March 11, representatives from the CBI Lab informed the Vistronix site supervisor that the initial test result of Thursday's mail sample would be delayed due to a preliminary positive test result. The Vistronix supervisor did not inform DoD of this preliminary test result. Over the weekend, CBI performed a confirmation test on the sample.

On Monday morning, March 14, at 6:15am, Vistronix released Thursday's mail to the Defense Post Office for distribution. Three hours later, the CBI Lab informed the Vistronix site supervisor that test results from one of the swab samples from Thursday's mail resulted in a positive response for anthrax.

The Defense Post Office was notified of the positive test result, immediately shut down their facility, and notified PFPA. In the two hours that followed, we established a secure perimeter around the RDF, notified Arlington County, and set up an incident command post integrating local and federal emergency response efforts. 236 employees from the RDF were evacuated to a nearby vacant building until they could be briefed, tested, issued precautionary treatment, and offered counseling services. We coordinated with other Pentagon distribution offices, identified all possible recipients of the morning mail, and deployed HAZMAT teams to these sites for additional swab sample tests.

Between 10am and 1pm, PFPA notified local, state and federal emergency response agencies of the potential biohazard incident through the Washington Area Warning System. By 1pm the Centers for Disease Control and Prevention, the Homeland Security Operations Center, and the Office of the Post Master General were all notified.

Arlington County Fire Department arrived at the Pentagon at 11:04am and the FBI was on the scene by 1:00pm. Over the next three days, Pentagon officials coordinated with local, state and federal health and law enforcement agencies to coordinate response and communication efforts.

At approximately 2:00pm, we were notified that a bio-alarm was set off in a mail distribution office in Skyline 5. An officer was dispatched and requested assistance from Fairfax County, who responded and took over incident command. It was later determined that the room in question did not have a biosensor or bio-alarm. The device was a biological air filtration hood and the alarm was a red light indicating an airflow restriction.

All subsequent tests returned negative and the Skyline complex and RDF reopened on Thursday, March 17. By Thursday, March 17, the DiLorenzo Clinic in the Pentagon tested more than 800 people through nasal swabs and provided three days of antibiotics. Daily communication occurred with Pentagon employees to keep them informed of progress.

INITIAL ASSESSMENT

As in any emergency, there were actions that went very well and procedures that need to be improved. Our initial after-action assessments identified some positive aspects of the collective Pentagon response to this incident. The Remote Delivery Facility, as designed, kept potentially harmful substances isolated from the large Pentagon population. We immediately identified and screened potentially contaminated employees. Within 3 hours, our organic HAZMAT team completed 130 tests of the mailroom and other suspected areas.

As a result of an interagency conference between DoD, Homeland Security, Health and Human Services, CDC, the FBI and local authorities, a decision was made to advise, counsel, and treat several hundred postal service employees who handled the mail prior to its delivery to the Pentagon.

Not everything transpired, as it should have. It took too long for the original contractor lab mail results to be processed and the contractor staff failed to follow mail release procedures. Additionally, there was no way to confirm that all local, state and federal agencies heard the Washington Area Warning System message. The event illustrated that incidents at high profile symbolic federal facilities become breaking news stories and are quickly perceived as national events.

CORRECTIVE ACTIONS

We have already taken major steps to address these issues. Since the suspected anthrax incident, PFPA has assumed responsibility for oversight of the mail screening process and testing the samples from the filters at our Pentagon Laboratory. The on-site lab provides a 24-hour response for positive initial screening (or presumptive test) of multiple threat agents. PFPA will ensure the mail is properly quarantined until the Pentagon Lab returns negative sample test results.

Revised notifications, both interagency and external, are in place for future chem./bio events. Our procedures for using the Washington Area Warning System now include a preamble with an emergency message stating the "who, what, where, and when" of the event. We will ensure that a response is received from appropriate agencies such as DHS, FBI and local counties. In 30 to 45 seconds the emergency message will be repeated.

In addition to a number of after action reviews, a thorough review and assessment of the DoD response to, and management of, the incidents is being conducted. DoD will receive a draft after-action report in 21 days and a final report within 45 days.

The Pentagon is fortunate to have excellent working relationships with Arlington and Fairfax County's fire and police departments. These working relationships were tested and proven on 9/11 and continue to improve as we participate in annual exercises.

Mr. Chairman, this concludes my prepared remarks. Thank you for the opportunity to speak and I will be happy to answer any questions that you or the Committee Members might have.

Mr. SHAYS. Thank you.

We will start out with Ms. Norton. We are going to try to get at the bottom of what is still not clear to me as to where mistakes were made.

You have you the floor for such time as you need it.

Ms. NORTON. Thank you very much, Mr. Chairman.

Mr. Burrus, I am going to ask you to have somebody go with me to V Street. I am going to ask Mr. Day in the same way. You know, he laid it on the workers. We were able to—if you will forgive me, cross-examination that we are dealing with an unairconditioned facility. I think I just want to go there. It looks as though we did get a promise to deal with that situation. Very, very troubling.

I would like to know from you whether this is the first time— were not V Street workers put on Cipro?

Mr. BURRUS. On which occasion?

Ms. NORTON. On this?

Mr. BURRUS. On the most recent one?

Ms. NORTON. Yes, on the most recent one.

Mr. BURRUS. Yes, they were offered Cipro.

Ms. NORTON. Was this the first time since the anthrax attack in 2001 that any postal workers in the United States have been on Cipro?

Mr. BURRUS. No, the employees at V Street. This is the second or third occasion since 2001. There have been other circumstances where those employees in that facility have been put on Cipro.

Ms. NORTON. Mr. Burrus, that is very troubling testimony to me. We know that at the time of the anthrax attack that Cipro was not a very nice medicine to have to take. We also know, if you keep taking something, it doesn't work, and yet, of course, we have heard from the last panel that there's no way to tell when there's a false positive, that is, simply saying something is negative doesn't make it negative.

That's why you heard a lot of cross-examination by the chairman and me on that; your own testimony reinforces that. We are going to have to get to the bottom of that, particularly given your testimony that, in V Street, we have already had three times where people have had to take Cipro, and I understand that all of these are false positives.

So, I mean, how many times are we going to expose workers to a very important, probably the only drug they could take, and when the real deal comes, and it's our job to see that it doesn't, then many of them would have been exposed over and over again to this antibiotic and perhaps it wouldn't work as well. That is very, very troubling.

I want to move to Mr. Jester. Mr. Jester, is it your view that what we were dealing with here, we know we were dealing with a contractor. We know it was a noncertified contractor. So perhaps I ought to ask you why the Pentagon, of all places, was using a noncertified contractor. We had testimony in the prior panel—that this contractor was, "outside of the Pentagon system." If you have a system, I assume that within your system they are certified. Is that true? Those who are within the Pentagon system are certified by CDC?

Mr. JESTER. We utilize the CDC protocols in our laboratories, but the laboratory, to answer your question—the laboratory, the CBI in Richmond, this contract was set up in November 2001, right after the incident on the Capitol, and the Pentagon quickly came to the conclusion they need to screen the mail, and they had a contract with Vistronix. Vistronix in turn subcontracted with CBI Laboratory.

That process remained in place until this recent incident. We recognize there were some problems with that process.

Ms. NORTON. Well, subcontract—you didn't contract—there was a subcontract that resulted with this particular contractor being the laboratory?

Mr. JESTER. Yes.

Ms. NORTON. Not the contractor you in fact had employed?

Mr. JESTER. No, ma'am. The CBI laboratory was under contract to Vistronix who was under contract to the Army to screen the mail. And Vistronix screened the mail and sent their samples to the CBI Lab, so they were a subcontractor.

Ms. NORTON. I see.

Mr. JESTER. We recognize some problems with this. The Army had the American Academy of Sciences come in and take a look at the process and equipment. And they recognized there needed to be some changes. In fact, about 2 months before this event, the Army had asked my organization to take a look at the oversight of the screening process. And when we did that, we would then eliminate the CBI Lab and use our own laboratory.

Ms. NORTON. So are you any longer using this contractor or subcontractor to do lab work for the Pentagon?

Mr. JESTER. Pardon?

Ms. NORTON. Are you any longer using——

Mr. JESTER. No, ma'am.

Ms. NORTON. So you are no longer using——

Mr. JESTER. We stopped using it from the day of the incident.

Ms. NORTON. Are you using a CDC certified contractor?

Mr. JESTER. We are using a laboratory that we have with the Pentagon. The protocols that we use there are developed by the Army in consultation with CDC. The laboratory we have at the Pentagon is simply what I call a first alert laboratory. If we get a positive sample there, and we do have a PCR test there, we will immediately notify the FBI, and the FBI would take custody of that sample and then take it to the laboratory of their choice, which would be, I am sure, LRN laboratory.

Ms. NORTON. I guess that's all right, since you said, I understand, the Pentagon has perhaps the best experience with anthrax, because you have the military experience on which initially we relied. I will most certainly ask that—so when you said in consultation with CDC, I have to assume that CDC, that's the same thing as CDC certified. Because that consultation would not have their sign off, if it is not the functional equivalent of the certification?

Mr. JESTER. I would have to find out. I don't think there's a sample of approval per se. They did work with the CDC, the Army.

Ms. NORTON. They shouldn't be throwing their name around unless there is in fact something like that.

Mr. JESTER. Yes, ma'am.

Ms. NORTON. So I think you ought to get—if you would simply transmit to the chair by way of letter.

Mr. JESTER. Yes, ma'am.

Ms. NORTON. What the CDC consultation connotes so that we can translate it, do—does the lab use CDC reagents?

Mr. JESTER. Pardon?

Ms. NORTON. Does the lab use CDC certified reagents?

Mr. JESTER. No, ma'am.

Ms. NORTON. No? We use the Army agents, the Army's agents.

Ms. NORTON. Again, you know, that's going to be fine with me so long as two branches of government, the two agencies agree.

Mr. JESTER. Yes, ma'am.

Ms. NORTON. I have respect for the work that the Army and the military has done long before September 11th on anthrax, so just so we are talking about the same thing. But, again, I think that the chairman needs to have that understanding in writing.

Let me tell you what really disturbs me and I guess the chairman when he opened this set of questions really got to the bottom of the core concern we have. We really are not interested, if you see how Mr. Shays goes at these hearings, which is not to ask a question, say got you and go on to the next one. We really are interested in finding out what happened particularly with respect to coordination so that this can kind of be a test that leads to remediation everywhere. We did not mean it as a test but it amounts to that.

Now, in this region we have a National Capital Region Coordinator. I know it because it was my amendment to the bill that resulted in the National Capital Region Coordinator. When it got to the Senate it was even expanded. The feeling in both bodies was that this was the target region of the country, and while everybody else should have some kind of coordination in the States, since Federal facilities were located for the most part here, that the Department of Homeland Security should actually pay for the Coordinator.

In all of this testimony, I have a hard time finding that Coordinator, and indeed, I can't figure out what the protocols are. So I'm going to try to break it down and not ask, you know, who struck John.

Let me just ask a straight-forward question. Were there, let's leave aside what there are now because if there's something here now that was not there, you can tell me about that in answering this question. Were there, I will call them protocols, you can call them a list, for purposes of everybody understanding what I am talking about, that said once there is an incident, contact one, then contact two, then contact three, that kind of thing, the simple ABC's if you prefer of what to do in case there is an incident involving anthrax? Is there something that says immediately tell the National Capital Region Coordinator. Is there something that says go to the local police or fire, then go to X, Y?

Remember we are dealing with somebody who may be anybody. There may be a worker who says there is some powder here, I don't know what to do. Well, is there a piece of paper that says every worker should go to his supervisor and the supervisor knows bingo, 1, 2, 3, 4, 5? All those people immediately know, then the information flows out and because the experts then know, the information then flows back as to what to do?

If I could ask anybody who knows if there is anything written down that would tell a worker then or would tell a worker now what the steps are, let us say from 1 to 10 about who to notify or, if you like, what to do.

Mr. BURRUS. The Postal Service does have such information that is distributed to employees. The level of distribution is certainly dependent upon the managers in thousands of facilities across the country, but the real problem is we interact with all of the other agencies as well as private entities and everybody has a different protocol. There is no universal protocol. The Postal Service has its own. The Department of Defense or the Army, the Navy is not required to follow the Postal Service protocol. They have their own. So where the two intersect, as they differ, they differ. The Postmaster General, the U.S. Postal Service will follow his protocol, not that of the U.S. Army.

Ms. NORTON. But on an anthrax incident.

Mr. BURRUS. Yes, even with anthrax.

Ms. NORTON. Everybody has a postal facility.

Mr. BURRUS. Everybody suspects that if anthrax is identified that its origin—the initial suspicion is its origin is the U.S. Postal Service, particularly if it is discovered in a mailroom, and there are hundreds of thousands of mailrooms scattered in private entities. So if they discover anthrax in the mailroom, the immediate suspicion is that its origin was the U.S. Postal Service. That independent entity will follow their protocol and it will differ from what is followed by the U.S. Postal Service.

So you have conflicting protocols. What happened in the Pentagon recently, the suspicion was it was a Postal Service initiated action. There were two different protocols that were in play and the media was in between.

Ms. NORTON. What protocols were in play?

Mr. BURRUS. The Postal Service.

Ms. NORTON. And who else?

Mr. BURRUS. The Department of Defense because the suspicion was the anthrax was identified as having not been initiated but identified in the Pentagon.

Ms. NORTON. Mr. Jester, was there anything in writing that indicated in this region what you should do in a Pentagon postal facility if there was a suspicion of anthrax in the facility? Was there anything in writing which I am calling a protocol, but it is anything in writing? You can call it what you want to.

Mr. JESTER. Yes, ma'am. We have what we call a concept of operations, CONOPS, and we have detailed concepts of operations both for chem, bio and radiological situations, and it details what you do in each of those events, what kinds of notification you make.

Ms. NORTON. Who is the first person you would notify in this region?

Mr. JESTER. Arlington County. They are our first responder. And then based on what we see we would be contacting the FBI.

Ms. NORTON. Who would be doing this contacting, the person in the facility?

Mr. JESTER. Our operations center. Let me back up a little bit. We train our employees in the building. We give them training. For example, we provide all of our employees with escape masks like they have here in the Capitol. To get that escape mask they must come to a training class where they are educated on the chemical, biological or radiological threat and what they should do. And they are also told on who they should contact. They contact our emergency number.

We also train our employees on evacuation procedures. We also have an ability from our operations center to communicate to all 20,000 computers within a minute to say what is going on and what people should do.

We exercise these procedures, these CONOPS that we have on the chemical, biological, radiological; we exercise these measures each year with Arlington County Fire Department. We have an exercise that's called "Gallant Fox." So there are procedures set up for employees on who to contact and who we should contact.

Ms. NORTON. I'm with you so far as your emergency responders are concerned, but as I look at your testimony between 10 and 1 you say "PFPA notified, local," the various parties. Then you say by 1 p.m. the Centers for Disease Control and Prevention, Homeland Security Operations, Postmaster General were all notified. That is between 10 and 1. By 1 that is 3 hours. I do not even see the National Capital Region Coordinator in here. Maybe somebody told him along the line. I do not see anybody who was responsible after the emergency responders were notified to then make sure that there was proper notification given all over, and in fact the Mayor of the District of Columbia and the county executives have all complained about confusion in response. And part of the problem I am having is I don't see that it has made any difference to have a Regional Coordinator paid by the Federal Government in this region, and I still don't know who is in charge of this operation once anthrax is suspected. There's no question if there's a fire, first call the fire department, and that is what you had here, but after that there may be something far larger going on and I am not clear from your testimony or the other testimony where it goes after the emergency responders are notified.

Mr. JESTER. Ma'am, what we do is we use what is called the Washington Area Warning System. It's an open telephone line. It's a system maintained by FEMA. When you pick up that telephone line and give a message, we gave it three times that day.

Ms. NORTON. That should mean everything in the whole region got it long before 1; that should mean instant notification if it's an open line.

Mr. JESTER. It was around 12, I don't know the exact time.

Ms. NORTON. Why did it take so long? If it was an open line why wasn't there an immediate response, Roger, or whatever you say.

Mr. JESTER. Our first issue is we're working with Arlington County. That's our first responder.

Ms. NORTON. I understand that. That's the first thing you have to do, and I will get to them in a minute. After that, since this may be an anthrax attack, there may be some reason to tell the Congress and the White House, there may be a reason to tell God knows who, I wouldn't know who, therefore I would want somebody in the Federal Government who knows who to know and all I'm trying to find out is after you call the emergency responders who should we look to for leadership on this issue so that everybody knows to relate to that person.

Mr. JESTER. We utilize the instant command system. We have a unified command. We follow the National Incident Management System on who is in charge of the event. The Washington warning system also goes to over 80 organizations.

Ms. NORTON. It was just pointed out, in your testimony, you say there is no way to confirm that all local, State and Federal agencies, this is what you've testified, heard the Washington Area Warning System message. So there's no way for them to say Roger, got you.

Mr. JESTER. There is no way of verifying.

Ms. NORTON. That isn't technology. That's what you could have done 100 years ago virtually. Mr. Jester, it is not you alone. We have a problem far larger than you. I'm just trying to figure out how it works.

Chief Schwartz, did you want to clarify how this communicating worked?

Chief SCHWARTZ. A couple of points. One is that the National Capital Region Coordinator is not an operational position. While his role is to assist——

Ms. NORTON. I'm fully aware of that but for him not to know, what's the point? Let's get rid of him them.

Chief SCHWARTZ. I'm getting to that. The way that the system is supposed to work is that initial notification and response is made, and then the jurisdiction in which the incident is occurring establishes their emergency management system. They may open their emergency operations center.

Ms. NORTON. Say that again. Who establishes?

Chief SCHWARTZ. The local jurisdiction. In this case, originally Arlington. When Fairfax had their incident they did the same thing. They are opening their local emergency operation center. That becomes the conduit from the incident scene, through the local jurisdiction, and possibly, and in this case this was done, to the State. The State is notified of the incident. It has an awareness for what's going on. The State, if they feel the need to notify the Federal Government, they can do that. Normally that occurs when we are requesting additional resources, when we are requesting something that is not available.

Ms. NORTON. Chief Schwartz, you are dealing with how a local official would normally through the chain of command up to his Governor handle this matter. But what we in Congress have to worry about is that anthrax is not a local or State concern. Once you are talking about anthrax you are immediately talking about a major Federal concern. You did the right thing. In fact, if anything the reports about Fairfax and Arlington or even D.C., which wasn't as closely involved, were that they responded appropriately. But anthrax is a national concern. It involves a Federal matter. And I cannot yet figure out after you did your job, which was making sure, one, that you got there, and, two, that you located everybody who should have been notified in your jurisdiction. Still the Federal Government is over here someplace where all the information and knowledge about how to deal with anthrax is supposed to reside and I can't find out who is in charge.

I don't know if it's DHS. I don't know if it's the Pentagon. I don't know if it's the National Capital Region Coordinator. I don't know if it's the Department of Homeland Security, somewhere in the bowels of that organization. I don't know if it is the Postal Service, which is a Federal agency. I don't know who Mr. Jester is supposed to relate to. He's just in one agency. And at this point I can't figure that any of you know as well.

Chief SCHWARTZ. The answer is it's the local authority. The Federal Government does not take control even of anthrax.

Ms. NORTON. But we are not talking about control. You see, I've got to make sure we understand what we're talking about.

Chief SCHWARTZ. Because the issue you're talking about is notification.

Ms. NORTON. I'm not talking about notification in the local or county sense.

Chief SCHWARTZ. I know but here's the point that I was going to make, and this touches on something that Mr. Jester just mentioned. There is no reliable system in the National Capital Region where a jurisdiction can make a notification about an incident and be assured that everybody who has a need to know in fact gets that information.

Ms. NORTON. That really is all I need to know. The fact is that Mr. Jester has testified that this Washington Area Warning System message open line was used. And yet he did not know, or he is not able to say in his testimony that such primary actors as the actual operation center, you are talking operation, he cannot say for sure. He can only say for sure that their operations center at Homeland Security knew by 1 p.m. We are talking about 10 a.m. when all of this began, whatever the local officials were doing. And all reports are they were doing—they handled their own internal protocols appropriately. What we can't understand is how the Federal Government was not itself coordinating its appropriate response.

Mr. Schaenman, you have looked at this matter in terms of the actors who were involved. As I have indicated, I'm not concerned about the emergency response because they have tested and rehearsed and they are just there when there is an event. But once they get there we are talking about anthrax. What in the world are they going to do? Anthrax has to go some place to be verified. Somebody has to say, I'm in charge here, everybody relate to me. And I would be very interested in what you found and where you think the flaws were, who you think might have been in charge or should have been in charge and what you'd recommend.

Mr. SCHAENMAN. Your question actually raises a whole bunch of issues. It's not a single simple thing. As the chief was saying, the actual incident was managed very well. There was unified command. In the face of uncertainty, the hard issue here was was it or wasn't it anthrax. So that drove a whole lot of things.

Ms. NORTON. Let me stop you there. So when the two chiefs go and the question is was there or was there not anthrax, what can they do? What can they do? Was it or was it not anthrax? What can two chiefs doing their jobs do?

Mr. SCHAENMAN. I think what happened early in the process, and, chiefs, tell me if this wasn't true, is the public health, the county level public health authorities get notified and start talking to each other and making medical decisions.

Ms. NORTON. Did your men and women go to the site?

Chief SCHWARTZ. Yes. To the Pentagon, yes.

Ms. NORTON. When you got there what could you do?

Chief SCHWARTZ. We immediately, recognizing the situation, notified our Office of Emergency Management. They operate our emergency management system. They have the connections throughout the local government. They immediately notified our local Public Health, who has a direct and statutory relationship to State Public Health because there is no Federal Public Health.

Ms. NORTON. What did they do about the substance or the part of the facility where it was thought that anthrax was suspected? What could they do about that? Here is where I'm trying to see the relationship between the Federal Government and the State authorities.

Chief SCHWARTZ. What they're doing is they're working with the folks on the ground, in this case at the Pentagon and I presume at the Fairfax facility also. They're working with Federal law enforcement personnel.

Ms. NORTON. Do either Fairfax or Arlington have facilities for testing?

Chief SCHWARTZ. No, we rely——

Ms. NORTON. No matter what you can't test.

Chief SCHWARTZ. We have some minimal field testing capabilities to give us some indication as to what we may be dealing with. That was not necessary here although there were a number of those tests done.

Ms. NORTON. Let me go to Mr. Schaenman and then I will go to the chairman, who has been very gracious. The point I have been trying to establish is that making their very best, even heroic efforts, when it comes to anthrax, local emergency responders are at the mercy of somebody who can test to see if there is anthrax. I don't care how good they are, that is not their job. That is why I'm interested in the relationship between the local responders here, two counties that acted appropriately, and what looks to be the only entity that can get at whether or not we have a homeland security emergency. And Mr. Schaenman and I know Chief Neuhard also wanted to say something on that. So I would like your responses.

Mr. SCHAENMAN. The information flowed very fast, very early. NCR did know about it. NCR did participate in disseminating waves of information. It was not the only route.

Ms. NORTON. So who was in charge?

Mr. SCHAENMAN. So the people in charge of the incident, dealing with the incident were the local authorities.

Ms. NORTON. Here we go again. I know that. I've just established they can't do anything. They don't know what it is. They are doing their jobs. Who's in charge of everybody here? They're fine, so is everybody else fine. Mr. Jester has done what he's supposed to do. He said he's talked on his little phone and said hey out there, anthrax, anthrax, but nobody answers him back because that's not a part of the protocol. That's what I'm trying to find out. Who is in charge, who should be in protocol?

Mr. SCHAENMAN. There's one set of protocols that deal with disseminating the information about an emergency. There's a different set of protocols that deal with dealing with the action. It goes into the public health sector. The public health people who are alerted at the local, State and national level, it was going in waves. So lots of people are readied, resources were being readied to move drugs but until the incident gets beyond the local governments it doesn't——

Ms. NORTON. Who's in charge, Mr. Schaenman, who's in charge?

Mr. SCHAENMAN. The local agencies are in charge. I mean, the incident commanders are in charge. There's a medical answer also.

Ms. NORTON. Well, that's certainly not acceptable. It's not that your answer isn't acceptable. It's truthful, but it's not unacceptable to us that local authorities are in charge of a major homeland security national event.

Yes, sir.

Chief NEUHARD. There are through the incident management system very clear lines of authority and through State law and Federal law. The problem is as that escalates, as we asked for increased resources, which we do. And in this case we would need resources, there are Federal authorities that have very specific authorities on that scene and they would come integrate with us and we ask them for assistance in certain areas.

We had two different incidents here with two different sets of problems. The problem became that while we knew at the incident scene who the Federal representatives were and what they were doing and how they integrated with the system, as you moved away from the incident site and the sample is taken to the lab, we knew where it was going, and the scientists within the Federal Government and the agencies within the Federal Government became to bear on the problem, it then was a question by the localities.

We know who the responsible agencies are here, but we've got a lot of people talking and confused with no single clear point of contact about where this information should come back to the locality. And you're exactly right, we are slaves to that and that is a problem.

The incident management system provides the answer to that, but that assumes that the plans that are in place identify who the lead authorities are in that case. At the local level and the State level it says for the type of emergency who is supposed to be there. And the national response plan, if operated, is supposed to define that as well.

Ms. NORTON. Who does it say is supposed to be there? Who does it say is supposed to be the lead authority in this region in the event of an anthrax incident of the kind we had at the Pentagon, for example?

Chief NEUHARD. I cannot answer that clearly for you, Ms. Norton. It will have to be asked to Federal authorities.

Ms. NORTON. The chairman says why not. If you don't know, Chief Neuhard, since you clearly understand what is supposed to be at your level it is because there is not clarity at the Federal level about who is in charge. I mean, if we have established nothing else here today, we have established that there is nobody in charge when there is an anthrax event, that there is plenty of information flowing, and that really scares me because information flowing from multiple sources is as confusing and perhaps more confusing than no information, and I think the way it began, Mr. Jester, was the right way to begin. But it seems to me that little fixes here could help. It began apparently with you using this Washington Area Warning System message. That message could have been received not only by everybody and may have been but by, quote, whoever is in charge. But the first thing to know is how do you report back that you have gotten it and how do you know that whoever is in charge, this mystery person, has gotten it, so that we know that all of the action that is then supposed to take place is then taking place. I'm assured that at some point it was, but everybody reported confusion, and that confusion begins and ends with no point of responsibility and accountability for an anthrax attack in this region, and that is something that we've simply got to straighten out.

Mr. Chairman, thank you very much.

Mr. SHAYS. Before I go to staff to ask some questions, Mr. Jester, are you involved with the anthrax vaccine program?

Mr. JESTER. No, sir.

Mr. SHAYS. So would the Force Protection Agency—define to me what the Director of the Pentagon Force Protection Agency means. You are in charge of the building?

Mr. JESTER. I'm in charge of the security for the Pentagon reservation and other DOD office buildings in the National Capital Region that are not military reservations; for example, leased commercial buildings around the metropolitan Washington area. We perform a function that is very similar to the U.S. Capitol Police at this location.

Mr. SHAYS. So in the end are you agreeing with Ms. Norton that we really don't know who is in charge of anthrax?

Mr. JESTER. No, sir. We are all guided by the National Incident Management System, which establishes a process on who is in charge——

Mr. SHAYS. If you don't agree then, don't tell me we all are. Tell me who is in charge.

Mr. JESTER. There is an incident commander. There is a process described in the National Incident Management System. It describes an incident.

Mr. SHAYS. Is there a person with a name that is in charge overall? Who is that person? I see two heads shaking.

Mr. JESTER. It would depend on the nature of the incident. It is scenario driven, whether it is a law enforcement incident or whether it's a fire/rescue incident or whether it is a public health incident.

Mr. SHAYS. Anthrax. We'll take anthrax. Who's in charge?

Mr. SCHAENMAN. The local public health director.

Mr. SHAYS. I don't believe the local public health director can go into the Pentagon and take charge. I don't believe it.

Chief SCHWARTZ. And one of the things that the State and local after action report does point to is the fact that the public health dimensions; that is, the release of prophylaxis for those employees, was not well coordinated.

Mr. SHAYS. You said "and" like you were going to give me some information. I said I don't believe that the public health director can in fact take charge, can take command in the Pentagon and you started to say "and." What does "and" have to do with it? Are you agreeing or disagreeing that's true? Do you think the public health director can take charge? Can she tell Rumsfeld what to do?

Chief SCHWARTZ. No. But I'm saying by NIMS and by the National Response Plan she is supposed to be able to.

Mr. SHAYS. OK. So in theory the national public health director has jurisdiction, except that we learn from Dr. Schafer that DOD has separate requirements and basically plays by separate rules. So what is the point of your telling me that the health director has jurisdiction and is in charge when in fact they haven't been in charge? They aren't in charge, and they probably never will be in charge.

Chief SCHWARTZ. Well, I think that things have changed a lot in the last couple of years, but I would also say with all due respect, sir, that's the purpose of these kinds of hearings is to get to the bottom of that and perhaps resolve some issues that we are unable to resolve.

Mr. SHAYS. I basically view you as the good guy here in the sense that you are trying to help us sort that issue out, and I appreciate it. But it just seems to me we could just have someone without 30 minutes of questioning, if someone could say what it is and we don't have to do this kind of probing. I'm wondering why we have to do this kind of probing.

The bottom line is nobody is in charge in essence or there is a real disagreement as to who's in charge or that everybody's in charge therefore nobody is in charge. I mean, that would start us in this process.

Mr. JESTER. From the standpoint of the Department of Defense, the Assistant Secretary of Defense for Health Affairs, Dr. Winkenwerder, was our immediate public official, and he's the one that made the decision. He contacted CDC right away to talk about what he was facing. He was facing a situation where he had a positive test even though it was flawed but it was not known at the time. He had mail that was there for 5 days and he had 236 employees that were very concerned for their safety. So he made that decision, he made the public health decision.

Mr. SHAYS. Let's just take what you said, Dr. Winkenwerder, he basically notified CDC. Did he notify the health director?

Mr. JESTER. The local health director? Arlington County Public Health Director?

Mr. SHAYS. I'm not going to help you out as to who that would be. Did he?

Mr. JESTER. He did not notify directly the Arlington County Health Director. He talked to them later in the day.

Mr. SHAYS. Let's stop right there. Chief Schwartz, you are telling me who's in charge?

Chief SCHWARTZ. I'm telling you by statute in Virginia the local public health director has that authority, including on the Pentagon reservation. Now that did not happen in this incident, but that doesn't diminish the fact that is the law in the State of Virginia.

Chief NEUHARD. Mr. Chairman, I would say that in our incident in Leesburg Pike that did occur.

Mr. SHAYS. What is that?

Chief NEUHARD. That did occur, where our Public Health Director was the incident commander, decided when that building was going to be opened again based on the information provided to her, decided whether prophylaxis was going to be given to other building occupants. Now if the DOD went beyond that with their people that was their business, but very clearly in that case it was clearly our Public Health Director that was in charge after our initial response.

I would also say that in past histories where we have had chemical releases in buildings that have been occupied by Federal agencies we have taken control and command of those buildings. The problem comes when you get to a facility that is federally owned and not leased, such—in our case such as the CIA. Then it is a Federal reservation and we do support their operations.

Mr. SHAYS. So in my lingo support means don't take control, you just help them?

Chief NEUHARD. In most cases that is correct, sir. If it is on their land under their control then we support their operations. If they are in a position where they are in State or local lands, we very clearly take command and control and introduce our particular response plans to that. The incident commander will be the lead. It's defined. And if I were at the CIA ultimately there would be a Federal person that would be the lead on that incident, even though I would be in a unified command structure and providing my services at that incident under the National Incident Management System.

Ms. NORTON. Mr. Chairman, that is fine and that is appropriate because we are talking about the difference between a Federal property where you are preempted if the Federal Government so desires. And this facility was just an ordinary office building, isn't that true, and there were other people in there even besides—the Pentagon facility was not a Federal facility, isn't that right? It was an office building?

Chief NEUHARD. Skyline was not a Federal facility.

Ms. NORTON. It was not a Federal facility. So you understand we are not talking about preempting the State government. Indeed, I have to tell you that the D.C. government here pretty much had a very central role here even though we were talking about a Federal facility. So nobody would preempt you in an ordinary office building in the State of Virginia. What concerns us is that, for example, as with September 11th, you could have these incidents breaking out all over, No. 1. And that is their modus operandi by the way. That is exactly what they try to do, what you know they did do on September 11th, at least when they were using airplanes as weapons. That's the first thing.

The second thing is that with a biological attack it is particularly important that at some level the Federal Government certify whether or not there has in fact—such an attack has occurred, every bit as much as if that attack had been on an office building owned by a developer in downtown Washington. At some point the Federal Government would have to assure us that a biological attack had or had not occurred. So really all that we are asking about when we say "is not in charge," is not preempting the State officials who know better than the Federal officials could possibly know what to do in their own jurisdictions, but making sure that as with our questioning about certified laboratories, and so forth, with the prior panel that we are assured that we are not under attack, because if we are under attack Virginia may be the site but it is the United States of America that is under attack. Therefore, somebody in the Federal sector, particularly where all the information is—yes, there's a lot of information in public health departments, but that's why you pay taxes, for the Federal Government to come to grips with all of this.

So I just wanted to make that distinction that I do not think the chairman or I are talking about preempting the State of Virginia and you acted absolutely appropriately, but we do think the Federal Government should have somehow understood its appropriate role.

Mr. SHAYS. I am having trouble understanding who's on first and who's on second. I'm trying to sort out if there was a fire at the Pentagon, would the local fire department do that or would that be the Pentagon that would deal with the fire and then they would call in and who would have command.

Chief SCHWARTZ. Mr. Chairman, we can reply September 11th again and the attack on the Pentagon. It was the local authority that had all command and control for that incident.

Mr. SHAYS. Do you agree with that?

Mr. JESTER. Yes, sir, he was the incident commander.

Mr. SHAYS. See, I can almost understand it in reverse. I can almost understand that if the Pentagon had its own force they would be in charge because it is localized and they would ultimately, whatever consequence is localized. But I begin to be very uneasy if the Pentagon acts like China within the United States and there is a break out of SARS—I'm using that as somewhat an absurd example, but a biological problem that could go well beyond the confines of the Pentagon.

Now I realize anthrax isn't contagious so it is not maybe the best analogy, but when it's a health issue I have a greater appreciation that it has to be more than the Pentagon that is involved, and what I am left with and I will leave this hearing with a weird feeling that we really don't know who's in charge and that's very unsettling to me. And no one here is basically telling me—in theory you are telling me, Chief, that it is the health director but in practice you said it isn't. So then I don't know who's in charge.

Chief SCHWARTZ. I have to say, Mr. Chairman, that I think that is only with regard to the Pentagon. This is the third incident of anthrax that we have experienced in the National Capital Region or the northern Virginia area since October 2001, November 2003, and a couple of weeks ago at the Pentagon, and we learn more each time we deal with these. I would submit that there is no kind of response that we deal with in this country with regard to terrorism where a systems approach to dealing with it is more required than a biological incident. There are not—because what I will tell you is when the incident is confined to a specific site it is very easy to determine what command and control system, what set of resources you're going to apply to that, how you reach out for that next set of resources.

In a biological incident that spans—that knows no jurisdictional boundaries, and even in an anthrax incident the ones we went through before caused difficulties because the people that work at the Pentagon work in Maryland, they work in the District and they work in Virginia.

Mr. SHAYS. So anthrax could still be on their clothes and they could carry it out?

Chief SCHWARTZ. Anthrax could be in all those jurisdictions and three different public health authorities might have to manage their components of that incident.

Mr. SHAYS. So let me just be clear. In this incident, the Health Director in the Pentagon did not take command?

Chief SCHWARTZ. Correct.

Mr. SHAYS. And was notified in the beginning, others were?

Chief SCHWARTZ. Our Public Health Director was notified very early because again the system works such that the first responders arrive on the scene, recognize the problem, reach back through our communications mechanisms to activate our emergency management system, our emergency managers say to Public Health this involves you, this is not the traditional public safety responders by themselves, you're involved here.

Mr. JESTER. In our operations center we have the Arlington County Deputy Police Chief, we have the Public Health Office, and we have the Office of Emergency Management, all within our office.

Mr. SHAYS. And who is in charge?

Mr. JESTER. From the public health standpoint? It was just the Secretary for Health Affairs. He made the decision on the issue of antibiotics. The decision about isolating the areas was done initially by my personnel. When the incident first occurs, we secure the location. We are in charge. And again it is scenario driven. We have many exercises and, like Jim said on September 11th, many times the Arlington County Fire Department is the incident commander, in fact in many cases are the incident commander. But in the National Response Plan it talks about incidents of national significance. And from our operation of this event, it was looked at as a local event. There was no decoration that we know of, that I know of where it was declared an incident of national significance, which would then have made DHS come in. If that declaration had been made, DHS would have had a leading control.

Mr. SHAYS. We are not talking about DHS. We're talking the director of health in the area. And even then we did not have—that person was not in charge. That's all.

Each of us are doing—I mean, if I got blamed for all the inefficiencies of Congress because I'm a Member of Congress I would be pretty unhappy, and I am not blaming any of you but where I have a little bit of lack of patience it just seems we could have described this scenario a lot sooner and not taken so long.

In the end we know there is a lack of knowledge of who is in charge, not in terms of theory but in practice, and I would also say even in theory I don't believe the Secretary of Defense believes that the Health Director is in charge. I don't believe that for a minute. I do not think there is anything that would indicate that DOD in general thinks that the Health Director is in charge. At any rate I don't even know where this hearing is going to go because I don't know if anybody is going to pay any attention. I think DOD is going to keep doing what it does.

I will just say, Mr. Jester, my sense of concern just goes back to hearings years and years ago when we were asking about the anthrax vaccine program. And we said the way we were doing it was an experimental drug and the courts said yes, it was an experimental drug and stopped doing it, but we basically court-martialed people. We saw people from the National Guard go out. And even though the court said this was illegal, the Pentagon basically said we do not care. We are going to keep going on.

So there is a lack of credibility when I hear the word "anthrax," whether it is vaccines or who's in charge here. I just think DOD is going to do whatever the hell it wants, and I don't think it's going to be in our Nation's best interest.

Mr. JESTER. Sir, I think except for the situation of public health, we've had September 11th, we've had other exercises there, we've had other incidents there, and we've always followed the National Incident Management System. We do not want to operate independently because we need our partners in the local communities.

Mr. SHAYS. I think it would be good to sit down with the Health Director.

Mr. JESTER. And we will. Like I said, there are things we felt that, well, there are some things we need to work on, and that's one of the areas that we have to have some discussions.

Mr. HALLORAN. Dr. Statzenbach, I just want to ask if you heard the CDC testimony in the first panel. Did they describe any of the research that you are advocating in your testimony? Did you hear that any of it was underway or planned?

Dr. STETZENBACH. It is my understanding that CDC is working with Dugway in an experimental room to do the very research that we published on a couple years ago.

Mr. HALLORAN. Twenty years ago?

Dr. STETZENBACH. No, no. We published a couple papers in 2004 using an experimental room where we released an anthrax simulant and tested different sampling methods. They are now moving forward with that research in Dugway.

Mr. HALLORAN. Replicating your research?

Dr. STETZENBACH. I don't know if they're doing simulants or they're doing the actual anthrax. That's something we can't do in my laboratory. But our lab started off with some of that work. We're currently not doing it now.

Mr. HALLORAN. Anything else that you heard that would meet— the research you're advocating, did you hear anything else that is planned or underway?

Dr. STETZENBACH. There's a tremendous amount of research that needs to be done. As I was listening to the gentlemen here, it struck me that we can't lose sight of the fact that all of these different groups have a different focus. The first responders as they're called to a scene their question is, is there a threat. The public health officials want to know if there has been exposure and a resulting adverse human health effect. Law enforcement wants to know who did it and how can they gather their forensic evidence. And ultimately EPA wants to know what the scope of the contamination is so that they can get it cleaned up.

Each of those different groups right now has a different sampling strategy and it is chaos when they all show up at the same place at the same time.

Mr. HALLORAN. And I would suggest that each of them has different information needs in time. Whereas a fire is happening now, this thing moves across time and space as it were. You know things later that you would like to know now, which leads me to the next question to the chiefs. In terms of handheld assays or field tests for anthrax or biological agents, what do you know about their capabilities now? What do you feel now? What are their limitations and what realistically would you like them to be able to do?

Chief SCHWARTZ. A higher level of reliability is what we're looking for. But as I mentioned in my testimony that I want to be real clear with, we are not using a handheld assay or any kind of field testing. We are not using any handheld devices, any field testing to make clinical decisions. What we are looking to do is just manage the public anxiety when we're confronted with an incident like this, and when we're dealing with that we're dealing with it by doing a threat assessment and in consultation with our public health authorities.

So we want higher levels of reliability but it is hard for me to imagine today a level of reliability or validity that would change that portion of the response. We're still going to be making tactical decisions as a part of our incident management structure and consulting with Public Health to make those clinical decisions.

Chief NEUHARD. As I mentioned in my testimony, we are very concerned about the reliability and the accuracy of what is available today on the market. We believe we need it and what we want from it is for us to say yes or no, it is present, and do that with probably 99 percent reliability.

Dr. STETZENBACH. And those data are not out there.

Chief NEUHARD. And they're not there and that's the problem. But to say that they are not needed, we go through incidents, we maintain people onsites, we go through emergency actions over time because we don't have that answer and that prolongs the anxiety of the community. It prolongs the use of resources and we need a method that will allow us to do that. Now we keep getting closer. The PCR is the closest thing we've got today, but it's expensive. It requires a lot of training and a lot of use, and we're hoping that some day there is a better technology.

Mr. HALLORAN. Just two more. Mr. Schaenman, who convened those conference calls with 80 people on them?

Mr. SCHAENMAN. Some of them were, they were convened by the Department of Homeland Security. NCR convened some of them. There were others that were convened by counties.

Mr. HALLORAN. What was the point? What did they hope to achieve?

Mr. SCHAENMAN. I think they were trying to inform everybody where things stood. It wasn't just one call. It was a series of calls, and people were occupied with the call and it would be time for the next call. And they weren't using technology that allowed people to identify somebody who wanted to ask a question. It was a good hearted "let's tell everybody what's going on." The pendulum has swung the other way, from everybody guarding information to too many people spreading information. And the kernel of the information not being clear as to what test are you talking about, what does it mean, what's the timestamp on it? Am I hearing the same thing three different ways? Is it a positive test? Is it a negative test? What's the interpretation?

So there was almost overcommunication in these incidents. And people have called, all the State and local governments we interview have called, as Ms. Norton was suggesting, for a clearer protocol of who is responsible for sending the information beyond the county or jurisdiction of origin where it first starts.

Mr. HALLORAN. Finally, Mr. Jester, it was described in an incident that local responders were coming up to a DOD facility and they did not know what technology was being used inside. They didn't even know that any technology was being used inside. Is that true elsewhere throughout this area? Can you tell us if it is getting better?

Mr. JESTER. You're talking about the Skyline 5 incident?

Mr. HALLORAN. Yes.

Mr. JESTER. We didn't know there was technology that was being used. It was purchased by the tenants in that office. They used it, told no one except themselves, and so it confused Fairfax County. It confused us.

Mr. HALLORAN. Was that the human error?

Mr. JESTER. I think what is happening is that offices are concerned for their safety and they see a lot of brochures and things around and salesmen go around and try to sell things to them, and they buy them probably carelessly. Hardware is no good without concept of operations. If there is a device in a building, you need to have someone who knows what they're doing, how to use it. There should be manuals there and they should be coordinated with their local responders.

Mr. HALLORAN. Assuming for a moment that's the outlier, can you assure the committee that in DOD facilities not run by a contractor with technology that you don't know about, that you have made proper liaison with local officials so they know what's there when they get there?

Mr. JESTER. As far as we know, but what we're going to need to do is go out and survey. We have to go around to every office and ask the question, do you have a device here and if you do where is it, what is it, and in most cases tell them to shut it down until we can find out what they have and whether it is worthwhile.

Mr. HALLORAN. Thank you.

Mr. SHAYS. I would like to do a UC, and put into the record a letter and support materials from Assistant Chief Alan Vickery of Seattle, WA Fire Department. Without objection, so ordered.

[The information referred to follows:]

Halloran, Larry

From:	Alan Vickery
Sent:	Friday, April 01, 2005 11:46 AM
To:	Halloran, Larry
Subject:	Biological Screening
Attachments:	Biological Agent Questionnaire.doc; Biological Agent Guidelines.doc

Chairman Christopher Shays,

There is a general misunderstanding, in certain federal agencies, of the capabilities of properly trained first responder HazMat Teams.

HHS has repeatedly tried to take the biological screening tools away from us and simply rely on the "National Lab System". I absolutely concur with definitive analysis being conducted in a laboratory setting, but must continue to emphasis the need for field tactical decisions to be guided by screening technology in the hands-of trained first responders.

When you have a "release" of a powder in a building with 2,000 occupants, decisions need to be made regarding the level of threat it presents to the occupants and the responders. Field screening is essential to make informed tactical decisions. The utilization of PCR technology, basic chemistry, IR spectrometry, and immoassays are appropriate screening tools to determine the level of threat.

We need better field screening technology for biological agents.

Any technology in the hands of untrained individuals can lead to inappropriate conclusions. Training on the technology, appropriate operating protocols and the utilization of multiple screening tools are appropriate tools to assist in making decisions.

My request is to placed increased emphasis on enhancing field screening tools as well as laboratory capabilities.

I am attaching the "Biological Agent Guidelines" utilized by the Seattle Fire Department.

All our Firefighter/HazMat Technicians are trained to NFPA 472 standards. Response to a suspected biological agent are interdisciplinary with law enforcement and public health.

Thank you,

Assistant Chief A.D. Vickery
Operations Division
Seattle Fire Department
301 Second Avenue South

4/1/2005

Seattle, WA 98104
Phone: 206.386.1489 or 206.386.1895
Fax: 206.233.2755

Unit 77 Guidelines

BIOLOGICAL AGENT GUIDELINES

Biological agents for use as weapons

Getting the most infectious and virulent culture for the seed stock is the greatest hurdle. Four avenues to the acquisition of a pathogenic seed culture exist:
- Natural sources
- Culture collections
- Various research laboratories and public health facilities
- Terrorists i.e. state sponsors or discontented employees of countries that maintain bio-warfare capability

To employ a natural killer as a weapon of war is theoretically an alarmingly straightforward concept. However, effectively harnessing Mother Nature's killing capability is easier said than done.

Terrorists will find several barriers on the road to an effective biological attack, including the difficulty in obtaining a lethal strain. Included are the complexities of establishing a stable manufacturing process; the challenge of purifying the agent and keeping it alive during dissemination; and the selection of the appropriate means for the target and agent.[1]

Biological agents can be prepared and used either in liquid or dry form. Procedures and equipment for preparing liquid biological agents are simple, but the resulting product is difficult to disseminate into small-particle effective aerosols. Conversely, procedures for producing dried biological agents are complex and require more sophisticated equipment, yet this product is readily disseminated by any number of crude devices.

What do they look like?

Responders should have some notion of what a biological warfare agent looks like; yet, taking the descriptions too literally can lead to severe consequences. Each agent can be processed differently, during which its appearance may change. With these restrictions in mind, a review of the general appearances of several types of agents follows:

Liquid agents have a viscosity that is much thicker than water and less thick than a light pancake syrup or something like whole milk. The color of liquid agents can vary significantly. Most bacterial agents derived from fermentation will be amber to brown colored, but opaque. Egg-derived liquid agents will be either the color of egg yolk, or slightly pink to red.

---

[1] The Chemical and Biological Terrorism Threat and the US Response – The Henry L. Stimson Center October 2000

Unit 77 Guidelines

Dried agents might have the consistency of bath powder. An ideal dry agent should have free-flowing properties. If the powder is derived from a highly-sophisticated process, it would contain very small particles (1 to 5 microns in diameter) and be highly charged with static electricity. These particles tend to cling to surfaces and are most difficult to handle. A less-sophisticated process yields a course-appearing powder which is composed of large particles (10 to 20 microns in diameter) and is not particularly difficult to handle.

The color of dried agent reflects the liquid from which it was derived; that is, dried bacterial agents tend to be amber to brown in color; viral agents derived from a tissue culture system will be an off-white; viral and rickettsial agents derived from embryonated chicken eggs will be either brown to yellow or pink to red. Unfortunately, these descriptions can be distorted by a smart adversary who can incorporate appropriate dyes into the suspension to be dried, and thus change everything.

How are they disseminated?

Terrorists are most likely to employ a liquid agent and disseminate it from a single-fluid device such as a garden sprayer or point sprayer. These devices, although readily available, are not efficient in generating a small-particle, highly infectious aerosol.

A dried agent with the desired properties requires serious development with skilled personnel and sophisticated equipment. The ABC fire extinguisher is a good example of such a system. Placed upwind of the intended target or at the air intake of a building, this device can produce a large number of infections.

Municipal water supplies are very difficult to contaminate to cause widespread causalities. Dilution and diffusion factors as well as chlorination combine to make this type of operation non-feasible.

Dermal exposure is not an effective means for the dissemination of biological weapons. Intact skin provides and excellent barrier for most, but not all, biological agents. Mucous membranes, damaged skin, or open wounds constitute potential breaches of the natural dermal barrier through which biological agents may pass.[2]

For maximum effectiveness, a biological agent must be delivered as an aerosol. An aerosol is defined as a suspension of finely divided liquid or solid particles suspended in a gaseous medium. Examples of common aerosols are mists, fog, and smoke. But not just any aerosol will work.

---

[2] Jane's Chem-Bio Handbook

Unit 77 Guidelines

To penetrate the lungs deeply enough to cause serious infection, the aerosol particles must be between one and five microns in diameter (one micron is one one-thousandth of a millimeter). The upper respiratory tract filters larger particles; smaller particles are unstable in ambient environmental conditions.

Detailed description of Anthrax[3]

Anthrax is a zoonotic disease caused by Bacillus anthracis. Under natural conditions, humans become infected by contact with infected animals or contaminated animal products. Human anthrax is usually manifested by cutaneous lesions. A biological warfare attack with anthrax spores delivered by aerosol would cause inhalation anthrax, an extraordinarily rare form of the naturally occurring disease.

The disease begins after an incubation period varying from 1-6 days, presumably dependent upon the dose of inhaled organisms, though in some cases, spores lodged in the lungs may take up to 60 days to germinate. Onset is gradual and nonspecific, with fever, malaise, and fatigue, sometimes in association with a nonproductive cough and mild chest discomfort. In some cases, there may be a short period of improvement. The initial symptoms are followed by 2-3 days by the abrupt development of severe respiratory distress with dyspnea, diaphoresis, stridor, and cyanosis. Once inside the body, anthrax bacteria emerge from their dormant spore phase and begin to reproduce and spew out toxins, which poison tissues and cause organs to fail. Inhaling spores is most likely to result in death because the germs burrow into lung tissue, where they come in close contact with lymph vessels. These serve as the body's liquid highway, transporting nutrients, debris and bacterial toxins throughout the body. Physical findings may include evidence of pleural effusions, edema of the chest wall, and meningitis. Shock and sudden death can occur within four hours of respiratory symptoms and fever onset.

If cases have been diagnosed, prophylaxis with ciprofloxacin, doxycycline or penicillin is recommended. Effectiveness of antibiotic use will depend on how early treatment is started and the antibiotic sensitivity of the organism. Anthrax is not transmitted from person to person. Case-fatality rate is high following onset of pulmonary signs and symptoms.

About 8,000 to 10,000 spores are typically required to cause pulmonary anthrax.[4]

ERP can be protected from anthrax spores by wearing splash protection, gloves, full face HEPA respirators or SCBA (Level C or B protection)[5]

---

[3] The Medical NBC Battlebook
[4] Jane's Chem-Bio Handbook
[5] Memorandum #50-99

Unit 77 Guidelines

Responding to an anthrax threat

A low-credibility threat is treated similar to a telephonic bomb threat. Initially, there is not obvious physical evidence to substantiate the threat. These incidents will require the dispatching of a single Fire Department Company to assist Police in evaluating the treat and if necessary implementing initial hazmat scene protocols of isolation, deny entry, evacuate, and call for assistance.[6]

When a determination is made that a credible threat exists (prior intelligence information, a suspicious envelope, package, or device, when physical evidence is found, or the release of an unknown substance has occurred), the incident will be treated as a crime scene involving hazardous materials. These incidents will require the dispatching of a hazardous materials response in addition to Police resources. Fire Department and Police Department resources will be coordinated to mitigate and investigate the incident.[7]

Company operations guidelines

- Upon arrival, establish command, give a comprehensive size-up and request additional resources if needed.
- Request Seattle Police if they have not been dispatched.
- Contact the responsible party.
- Isolate and deny entry. Immediately limit the number of civilian and uniformed personnel exposed to the hazmat by identifying and establishing an isolation perimeter – the initial Hot Zone.
- Control building's operating systems such as the HVAC, elevators, fire control panel, etc.
- Potentially contaminated patients do not need to be quarantined but should be encouraged to wash hands and face with soap and water.
- Complete as much of the Biological Agent Questionnaire as possible. Do not risk exposure – the subjection of a crew-member or yourself to the hazmat through any route of entry i.e. inhalation, ingestion, skin absorption, or direct contact.
- If possible, list the names and telephone numbers for all people who were in the room or vicinity where the material was found.
- Wait for the Reconnaissance Team (Recon 1) or Hazardous Materials Response Unit (Unit 77).

---

[6] Memorandum 163-01
[7] Memorandum 163-01

Unit 77 Guidelines

<u>Hazardous Materials Unit – Reconnaissance Team (Recon 1)</u>

Team of 8 members (1-7) that will be dispatched to incidents that involve prior intelligence information, a suspicious envelope, package, or device, when physical evidence is found, or the release of an unknown substance has occurred to determine the validity of the incident. An Engine Company + a Battalion Chief will also be included.

Entry and Back-up Team members shall don Level B protection for the majority of their activities. Members performing field testing shall also don Level B protection.

In some cases, ERP may use a full facepiece respirator with a <u>P100</u> filter or powered air-purifying respirator (PAPR) with high efficiency particulate air (HEPA) filters <u>when it can be determined</u> that an aerosol-generating device was not used to create high airborne concentrations, and the dissemination was by a letter or package that can be easily bagged. [8]

Structural firefighting gear with SCBA may be utilized for those hazards that are flammable or combustible.

Team members will either validate or reject the incident as credible based on what they see or sense.
- Situations with higher credibility are those with a distinct threatening message included with the material, letter or package.
- Situations with lower credibility are those without a message or when it is an expected letter or package that is easily traced to the sender.
- If they chose to reject the incident as being credible they should have conclusive reasoning for their decision.
- If they chose to validate the incident as credible, a Hazardous Materials Response shall be requested.

In either case, the Recon Team shall:
- Contact the responsible party for the premises or the reporting party.
- Assess the need to control building operating systems (HVAC, elevators, fire control panel, etc.).
- Isolate and deny entry the potentially contaminated area. This area shall be their initial Hot Zone.
- Conduct evacuation to secure area and isolate potentially contaminated patients elsewhere.
- Secure and contain the product.
- Establish decontamination areas as needed.

---

[8] Interim Recommendations for Firefighters and Other First Responders for the Selection and Use of Protective Clothing and Respirators Against Biological Agents – Centers for Disease Control and Prevention

Unit 77 Guidelines

- Equipment choices:
  1. Sampling kit
  2. HazCat kit
  3. Ludlum – Radiological
  4. Exploranium GRC-135
  5. RadSmart
  6. MESO Systems BioCapture, Guardian BTA Reader & Tetracore test strip – Saphylococcus Enterotoxin B (SEB), Anthrax, Ricin, Botulism, Yersinia Pestis plague and Tularemia
  7. Drager CDS kit – Sarin, Tabun, Soman, Mustard, Lewisite, Hydrogen Cyanide, Cyanogen Chloride, and Phosgene
  8. Drager CMS kit – Phosgene, Chlorine, and knowns
  9. JenPrime PrimeAlert – Powder Screen Test Kit and Toxin Test Kit
  10. 20/20 Powder Test Kit
  11. Sensidyne Polytech 4-tube manifold – Chlorine, unknown organics and inorganics
  12. M8 paper – Sarin, Tabun, V-Agent, Soman, Mustard, and Lewisite
  13. M9 tape – Sarin, Tabun, V-Agent, Soman, and Lewisite
  14. M256A1 kit – Sarin, Tabun, V-Agent, Soman, Mustard, Lewisite, Hydrogen Cyanide, Cyanogen Chloride, and Cyanide
  15. ppb RAE – Chlorine and knowns
  16. Mini RAE 2000 – Chlorine and knowns
  17. Multi RAE Plus – Chlorine and knowns
  18. APD 2000 – Sarin, Tabun, V-Agent, Soman, Mustard, and Lewisite
  19. MSA Passport CGI
- Establish and maintain communications link with potentially exposed individuals.

Hazardous Materials Response Unit (Unit 77)

Unit 77 shall provide the following:
- Establish initial control zones.
- Establish decontamination area.
- Contact Chief Vickery at 206-386-1895, 206-200-7845 cell, 888-788-1298 pager
- HazMat Team Leader or HazMat Team Safety should contact the following:
  - Seattle Police Bomb Squad if they have not been notified (Sgt. Jim Hansen 206-255-7595)
  - FBI Designated Coordinator for WMD Jim Keesling 206-262-2055 (office), 206-622-0460 (24-hour), 206-559-1321 (pager). Note: SPD will also contact the FBI, so this call is optional.
  - Washington State Public Health Laboratory 1-877-539-4344 (a 24-hour emergency phone number) if testing is imminent.
  - Seattle/King County Public Health Duty Officer 206-296-4606
- Complete the information on the Biological Agent Questionnaire.
- Complete chain-of-evidence for sample.

- Confirm or rule out agent using the following equipment:
  1. Sampling kit
  2. HazCat kit
  3. Ludlum – Radiological
  4. Exploraniun GRC 135
  5. RadSmart
  6. MESO Systems BioCapture, Guardian BTA Reader & Tetracore test strip – Saphylococcus Enterotoxin B (SEB), Anthrax, Ricin, Botulism, Yersinia Pestis plague and Tularemia
  7. SensIR Technologies *TravelIR*™ HCl HazMat Chemical Identifier – Sarin, Tabun, V-Agent, Soman, Mustard. Note this unit <u>will not</u> identify biological agents
  8. Drager CDS kit – Sarin, Tabun, Soman, Mustard, Lewisite, Hydrogen Cyanide, Cyanogen Chloride, Phosgene
  9. Drager CMS kit – Phosgene, Chlorine, Knowns
  10. JenPrime PrimeAlert – Powder Screen Kit and Toxin Test Kit
  11. 20/20 Powder Test Kit
  12. Sensidyne Polytech 4-tube manifold – Chlorine, Unknown organic & inorganic
  13. M8 paper – Sarin, Tabun, V-Agent, Soman, Mustard, Lewisite
  14. M9 tape – Sarin, Tabun, V-Agent, Soman, Lewisite
  15. M256A1 kit – Sarin, Tabun, V-Agent, Soman, Mustard, Lewisite, Hydrogen Cyanide, Cyanogen Chloride, Cyanide
  16. ppb RAE – Chlorine, Knowns
  17. Mini RAE 2000 – Chlorine, Knowns
  18. Muti RAE Plus – Chlorine, Knowns
  19. APD 2000 – Sarin, Tabun, V-Agent, Soman, Mustard, Lewisite
  20. MSA Passport CGI

Hazardous Materials Response Unit's Field Screening Tests

SensIR Technologies Travel*IR*™ HCl HazMat Chemical Identifier

The Travel*IR*™ HCl identifies solids and liquids quickly and reliably, however it <u>will not</u> identify a biological agent. Its use will be in confirming that the product is something other than biological i.e. sugar, drywall compound, etc.

The Matt Fox HazCat Organic/Biological Hazard Test

The HazCat steps are as follows to test for organics on unknown solids; See flow chart for unknown solids in the HazCat procedures.

If the unknown solid appears inert, go to the oxidizer/acid test. If not inert, return to the flow chart.

Unit 77 Guidelines

- Oxidizer/acid test

Place a small amount of acid test on the test dish and a small amount of the unknown solid into the acid test. Observe reaction. Choose the most appropriate option.
  - If there is a reaction on the oxidizer test paper, then the solid is not a biological.
  - If there is no reaction, go to the water solubility test.
  - If there is another type of reaction, return to the flow chart.

- Water solubility test

Place ½-inch of water in the test tube. Place a small amount of the unknown solid into the tube with the water. Observe reaction.
  - If the unknown solid floats, add detergent to release the surface tension.
  - If it sinks at any time, the unknown solid is inorganic and not biological.
  - If it dissolves without residue, it is probably not biological.
  - If it sinks, suspends, or in part dissolves, go to the hexane and alcohol solubility test to determine if it is affected by polar or non-polar solvent.
  - If it floats after detergent is added, perform the char test.

- Char test

Place a small amount of the unknown solid into a test tube (approximately ¼-inch). Light torch. Holding the test tube in a wire holder, gently heat the bottom of the tube. Try to light off gassing material. Observe reaction.
  - If there is charring similar to cigarette ash, then unknown solid <u>is a possible</u> organic/biological. Make decision as to test or not to test using Tetracore BTA test strip.
  - If there is no reaction, sublimation, or tarring, then the unknown solid is <u>not</u> organic/biological.

If the field tests conducted thus far indicate that the product is possibly an organic/biological and additional tests are required at the Public Health Laboratory, the following shall apply:
- Packaging for transportation must meet the following criteria:
  1. All specimens that meet the criteria for submission must be coordinated with the Public Health Laboratory by calling 1-877-539-4344 a 24-hour emergency phone number.
  2. Any specimens other than dry powder or paper material must be screened for <u>radiological, chemical, or explosive materials</u> before it can be processed by the Washington State Department of Health Public Health Laboratory.

Unit 77 Guidelines

Field Screening for Radiological, Chemical, or Explosive Materials

- Radiological – Ludlum survey meter
- The Scott Marcus Life Safety Test
- Explosives – request SPD Bomb Squad to x-ray

The Scott Marcus Life Safety Test

- ### Reactivity Test (hairpin test)

  Objective: Conducted to test product (solid or liquid) for explosiveness and reactivity.

  Procedure:
  1. Heat hairpin until end is red-hot!
  2. Touch red-hot pin to product.
  3. Observe reaction – be prepared for a violent reaction!

  Conclusion:
  1. Is product reactive or not?

- ### Ignitability Test

  Objective: Conducted to test product (solid or liquid) for flammability/combustibility.

  Procedure:
  1. Light match away from product.
  2. Bring match to edge of watch glass and move inward toward product.
  3. Observe when and if product ignites.

  Conclusion:
  1. Ignition at edge of watch glass = very flammable.
  2. Ignition over product = flammable.
  3. Ignition when dropped in product = combustible.
  4. No ignition = not flammable or combustible.

- ### Oxidizer Test

  Objective: Conducted to test product (solid or liquid) for corrosivity.

  Procedure:
  1. Take a potassium iodide test strip and put 2-3 drops of 3N HCL on it.
  2. Drop it on the product.
  3. Observe the reaction.

Unit 77 Guidelines

Conclusion:
1. Strip turns black to purple and back to white rapidly = strong oxidizer.
2. Strip turns black slowly = weak oxidizer.
3. No change to strip = not an oxidizer.

- ph Test

Objective: Conducted to determine if product is acidic or basic.

Procedure:
1. Take pH test strip and dip into product.
2. Compare results with pH container.

Conclusion:
1. 0 through 6 = acidic.
2. 7 is neutral.
3. 8 through 14 = basic.

- Peroxide Test

Objective: Conducted to test product (solid or liquid) for peroxides to determine if they are potentially explosive.

Procedure:
1. Take peroxide paper and place a drop of water on it.
2. Touch paper to product.
3. Observe the reaction.

Conclusion:
1. If paper turns blue = product contains peroxides and is potentially explosive!

To provide a consistent message to the public regarding the outcome of our field screening, we should use the following language:
- If our field screening indicates that the product is an inorganic substance – not hazardous our statement would be *inorganic substance – not hazardous.*
- If our field screening indicates that the product is an organic and a possible biological, but the BTA test indicates negative our statement would be *organic substance, inconclusive and the citizen may call King County Public Health at 206-296-4949.*
- If our field screening indicates that the product is an organic and a possible biological, and the BTA test strip indicates positive our statement would be *organic substance, inconclusive and the citizen should be encouraged to call King County Public Health at 206-296-4949.*

Unit 77 Guidelines

- The following statements should not be used:
  - *See your doctor.*
  - *The test was negative for anthrax...*
  - *The test was positive for anthrax...*[9]

If there is not enough product to conduct the two field screening tests (1/2 to 1 tablespoon) but you decide to conduct a test using one or more BTA test strip(s) then the test strip(s) as well as the materials used to conduct the test shall be sent to the Public Health Lab for them to analyze. Even though our BTA test strip may indicate a negative test, there may be trace amounts of a hazardous biological agent that the test failed to pick up.

Packaging for transportation must meet the following criteria:

1. Place the specimen in a plastic zip-lock bag, wipe the outside of the bag with a solution of 9 parts water and 1 part bleach, and label biohazard.
2. Place the zip-lock bag into a leak-proof container with a tight cover and label biohazard.
3. Place this container into a second leak-proof container with a tight cover and label biohazard. The size of the second container should be no larger than a one-gallon paint can.
4. Place the second container into a third leak-proof container with a tight cover and label biohazard. The size of the third container should be no larger than a five-gallon paint can.[10]
5. Note: any letter or communication which threatens the presence of smallpox must be sent directly to the Centers for Disease Control and Prevention (CDC) for analysis, after being packaged.[11]
6. Note: A letter containing a powder which threatens the presence of anthrax must be sent to a member of the Laboratory Response Network.[12]

Hazardous Materials Response Unit

- Specific information to be documented when taking a sample:
  1. Location the sample was taken from.
  2. Time and date.
  3. Name of member(s) who took sample.
  4. Names of member(s) who handled sample.
  5. Other pertinent information.

- Decontaminate exposed individuals with soap and water. For anthrax, potentially contaminated patients do not need to be quarantined, nor placed

---

[9] Memorandum titled "Unknown Substance Incidents dated October 26, 2001
[10] Washington State Department of Health Public Health Laboratories Specimen Packaging and Transport Protocol for Suspected Bio-Terrorism Incidents
[11] FBI Intelligence Bulletin No. 32 – October 2, 2002
[12] FBI Intelligence Bulletin No. 32 – October 2, 2002

Unit 77 Guidelines

on chemoprophylaxis while waiting laboratory results. These patients need to be instructed that if they become symptomatic before laboratory results are available (usually within 48 hours), they should contact the Seattle-King County Health Department at 206-296-4949.

The disease begins after an incubation period varying from 1-6 days, though in some cases, spores lodged in the lungs may take up to 60 days to germinate. Onset is gradual and nonspecific, with fever, malaise, and fatigue, sometimes in association with a nonproductive cough and mild chest discomfort. In some cases, there may be a short period of improvement. The initial symptoms are followed by 2-3 days by the abrupt development of severe respiratory distress with dyspnea, diaphoresis, stridor, and cyanosis.

If cases have been diagnosed, prophylaxis with ciprofloxacin, doxycycline or penicillin is recommended. Effectiveness of antibiotic use will depend on how early treatment is started and the antibiotic sensitivity of the organism. Anthrax is not transmitted from person to person. Case-fatality rate is high following onset of pulmonary signs and symptoms.

- Treat exposed individuals. All potentially exposed individuals should be logged for later contact if needed. Distribute Follow-up Cards to these individuals.
- Those transporting exposed individuals shall contact the HMC ER Charge Nurse at 206-731-4025 to let them know patients are coming.
- Secure evidence & crime scene.
- Thoroughly document entire incident.

Mr. SHAYS. I would like to thank Bill Womack of Mr. Davis's legislative staff for very valuable help preparing for this hearing.

I would like to thank the patient and wide awake court reporters. Thank you very much.

I would also like to thank Kristine Kathleen McElroy of my staff, who has worked on this hearing, and to say that by the time the court reporter gives us the transcript her name will be Kristine Kathleen Fiorentino. McElroy is going to be history and it will be Fiorentino. Congratulations on your wedding next week.

Without any more important business to do, let us adjourn.

[Whereupon, at 6:05 p.m., the subcommittee was adjourned.]

[Additional information submitted for the hearing record follows:]

Submission for the Record
April 5, 2005
National Security Subcommittee Hearing on Addressing Anthrax Detection Methods

Response of **Dr. Klaus Schafer**
Deputy Assistant to the Secretary of Defense for Chemical and Biological Defense
Department of Defense

DoD Chemical Warfare Agent Confirmatory capabilities:

Fixed facility laboratories who can conduct confirmatory testing of Chemical Warfare Agents Using Validated and Standardized methods:

Edgewood Chemical Biological Center (ECBC)
Western Test Center Dugway Proving Ground
US Army Medical Institute for Chemical Defense

In addition there are several mobile assets that have laboratory equipment (Gas Chromatography-Mass Spectrometers, and Spectrophotometers) that can deploy to or near an incident and provide analysis that use validated and standardized laboratory procedures for identification, confirmation and quantization. These include:

ECBC
National Guard Civil Support Teams (CST) currently 32 certified CSTs operating with 55 teams to be certified and fielded by 2007.
U.S.M.C. Chemical Biological Rapid Response Force (CBIRF)
22nd Chemical Battalion (Technical Escort)
Air Force Institute of Occupational Health
Navy Forward Deployable Preventative Medicine Units (6 units)

Also, in the private sector the Battelle Columbus Medical Evaluation Research Facility that has the same capability as the three fixed DoD laboratories to conduct confirmatory testing of Chemical Warfare agents.

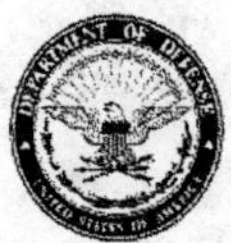
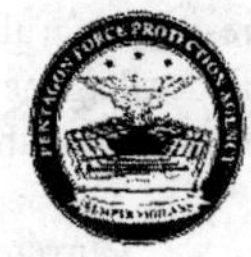

DEPARTMENT OF DEFENSE
PENTAGON FORCE PROTECTION AGENCY
9000 DEFENSE PENTAGON
WASHINGTON, DC 20301-9000

2 6 APR 2005

The Honorable Christopher Shays, Chair
Subcommittee on National Security, Emerging Threats, and International Relations
U.S. House of Representatives
B-372 Rayburn House Office Building
Washington, D.C. 20515

Dear Mr. Chairman:

Thank you for the opportunity to testify at your hearing on Assessing Anthrax Detection Methods. At the request of Delegate Eleanor Holmes Norton, I promised to get back to you to clarify the Pentagon Force Protection Agency's (PFPA) coordination with the Centers for Disease Control (CDC) in the stand-up of the new PFPA Pentagon Laboratory and in the type of reagents used.

There are currently no official certifications from the CDC for the protocols used in the new PFPA Pentagon Laboratory and for the corresponding reagents that are used. However, protocols and procedures used by the laboratory have been rigorously examined and qualified by the US Army Medical Research Institute of Infectious Diseases (USAMRIID) and the Naval Medical Research Center (NMRC). The CDC has recognized both USAMRIID and NMRC laboratories as definitive national laboratories within the Laboratory Response Network (LRN). In fact, reagents and protocols developed by USAMRIID have been adopted by CDC's LRN and the NMRC is an official member of the LRN. Additionally, the USAMRIID and NMRC certification authorities are derived from the LRN model where national-level laboratories certify that subordinate capabilities are qualified.

The PFPA Pentagon Laboratory is part of an analytical laboratory system under the Department of Defense (DoD) Chemical and Biological Defense Program. Early on, DoD established a laboratory testing quality assurance program within this analytical laboratory system. Laboratory operations meet all relevant local, state and Federal guidance and/or regulations. This rigorous quality assurance program evaluates each lab's technical performance and accuracy and assures comparability between laboratories by conducting blinded (unbiased) inter-laboratory comparative testing.

The reagents used by the PFPA Pentagon Laboratory are acquired from the Army and made available through the Critical Reagents Program (CRP). This program is administered through the Joint Program Executive Office for Chem-Bio Defense and has the mission of producing the highest quality detection reagents to serve as a national

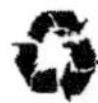

resource for the biological defense community. The CRP is actively working with other Federal agencies to create a nationally accepted process for standardizing how reagents, tests and methods are validated and utilized.

Currently, the PFPA Pentagon Laboratory is performing routine aerosol sample analysis. It is designed to be a high throughput, high confidence, environmental screening laboratory. It employs protocols for a variety of indoor/outdoor environmental samples, such as suspicious powders and liquids. Upon detection of a pathogen, the suspect sample will be referred to the FBI, who will send it for further testing to USAMRIID, NMRC, or another laboratory for a definitive sample analysis. This coordination with the FBI is consistent with procedures in the National Response Plan.

Under the auspices of an interagency Memorandum of Understanding on Coordinated Monitoring of Biological Threat Agents, the Department is actively working with the Department of Homeland Security, the Department of Health and Human Services, the Department of Justice, and the U.S. Postal Service to develop and implement a plan for an integrated national monitoring system. This new system will standardize laboratory protocols such as sample collection, testing, reporting and response.

PFPA is continuing to look at the CBRN programs for DoD offices in the National Capital Region and are working with State and local officials to improve communications in the event an incident similar to that of 14 March occurs. I hope this answers your questions. If you require further information, please do not hesitate to contact Colonel Armando Lopez at 703-614-2559 or me personally at 703-693-3685.

Sincerely,

John N. Jester
Director

Submission for the Record
April 5, 2005
National Security Subcommittee Hearing on Addressing
Anthrax Detection Methods

Response of Dana Tulis
Deputy Director for the Office of Emergency Management
Environmental Protection Agency

Monday, June 27, 2005 3:20 PM
Information for Subcommittee on National Security

The numbers were 22 out of 23 locations.

During the U.S. Capitol response, U.S. EPA initially
established a site characterization program at the Hart
building using 2-phase sampling approach. The first phase
(targeted sampling) was to collect samples in locations
most likely to have been contaminated by logical
contamination pathways (i.e. follow the mail, follow
people, follow the air). The second phase (statistically-
based) was to collect a large number of random samples
throughout the building. After both sampling phases, 23
discrete locations were identified as contaminated. Of
those 23 location, only 1 was identified via random
sampling - the other 22 were located by targeted
strategies. It is important to note that although we used
statistical methods to do this (e.g. collected random
samples over and evenly spaced areas); because we don't
know sampling efficiencies (e.g. validate the methods) or
have risk-based criteria for cleanup (based on validated
methods), it is impossible to calculate the probabilities
(which was GAO's recommendation) based on these
statistically-based techniques.

To put it simply, if we're only looking for one spore, we'd
have to collect samples over 100% of the surfaces and
through the volume of air.

One more thing... we don't have the files from the U.S.
Capitol Incident. They were turned over to the U.S.
Capitol Police.

Holly Smithson/DC/USEPA/US@EPA

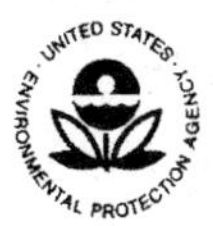

UNITED STATES ENVIRONMENTAL PROTECTION AGENCY
WASHINGTON, D.C. 20460

DEC 3 2004

OFFICE OF CONGRESSIONAL AND
INTERGOVERNMENTAL RELATIONS

The Honorable Christopher Shays
U.S. House of Representatives
Washington, DC 20515

Dear Chairman Shays:

Thank you for your letter of October 28, 2004, to Administrator Leavitt concerning the follow up from the October 28, 2003, hearing before the House Government Reform Committee, Subcommittee on National Security, Emerging Threats and International Relations.

We have provided a response to Congressman Nadler which addresses the concerns he raised at the hearing regarding the legal authority of EPA to act in the event of a terrorist attack (enclosed).

Again, thank you for your letter. If you have further questions, please contact me or your staff may contact Carolyn Levine, in EPA's Office of Congressional and Intergovernmental Relations, at (202) 564-1859.

Sincerely,

Charles L. Ingebretson
Associate Administrator

Enclosure

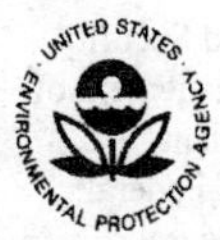

UNITED STATES ENVIRONMENTAL PROTECTION AGENCY
WASHINGTON, D.C. 20460

DEC - 3 2004

OFFICE OF
GENERAL COUNSEL

The Honorable Jerrold Nadler
U.S. House of Representatives
Washington, DC 20515

Dear Congressman Nadler:

I have been asked to respond to your question to Dr. Paul Gilman, former Assistant Administrator for the Environmental Protection Agency's (EPA) Office of Research and Development, during the October 28, 2003, hearing before the House Government Reform Committee, Subcommittee on National Security, Emerging Threats and International Relations, concerning the Environmental Protection Agency's legal authority to act in the event of a terrorist attack. I apologize for the delay in responding to you. We appreciate your continued interest in matters relating to lower Manhattan following the September 11th terrorist attacks.

Specifically, at the hearing you asked whether, in the event of a terrorist attack, it is EPA's responsibility pursuant to the Comprehensive Environmental Response, Compensation, and Liability Act (CERCLA) or Presidential Decision Directive 62 (PDD 62) to ensure the cleanup of releases of hazardous substances.

With respect to the EPA's authority under CERCLA, EPA is authorized under a variety of circumstances to respond to releases or substantial threats of releases of hazardous substances. The statute provides that the EPA is to give primary attention to those releases that may present a public health threat. Accordingly, EPA has considerable discretion in fashioning a response that will address the particular circumstance and the potential risk to the public.[1] If necessary, this authority can be used to address hazardous substances released to the environment by a terrorist attack.

---

[1] Responses to releases and substantial threats of releases are carried out under the National Oil and Hazardous Substance Pollution Contingency Plan (NCP). While the NCP gives EPA broad authorities to address the release and threat of release of hazardous substances, the NCP expressly states "[a]ctivities by the federal and state governments in implementing [the NCP] are discretionary governmental functions." The NCP "does not create in any private party a right to federal response or enforcement action [nor does it] create any duty of the federal government to take any response action at any particular time." 40 C.F.R § 300.400(i)(3).

Operating in concert with PDD 62 (discussed immediately below) is Homeland Security Presidential Directive (HSPD) 5, promulgated February 28, 2003, concerning the management of domestic incidents. Under HSPD-5 response to terrorism events is referred to as incident management. HSPD-5 provides, "the Secretary of Homeland Security is the principal Federal official for domestic incident management" and "the Secretary shall coordinate the Federal Government's resources utilized in response to or recovery from terrorist attacks, major disasters, or other emergencies." HSPD-5 also directed the Secretary to develop a National Incident Management System (NIMS), which provides a nationwide system for coordinating response and recovery efforts, and the National Response Plan (NRP), which integrates all Federal Government preparedness, response and recovery plans into a single all-hazards plan.

PDD 62, promulgated May 22, 1998, provides the general framework that governs the coordination of federal agency actions in the event of a terrorist attack, including an attack that involves the release or threat of release of a hazardous substance.[2] PDD 62 provides that "FEMA, the Lead Federal Agency for consequence management, is responsible for preparing for and responding to the consequences of a [weapon of mass destruction] incident with the participation of other departments and agencies including the . . . Environmental Protection Agency . . ., as necessary." Thus, while PDD 62 continues to exist, the NRP will provide the organizing structure for an EPA response.

Therefore, in the event of a terrorist attack, EPA would respond under the NRP pursuant to the annex entitled "Emergency Support Function (ESF) 10, Hazardous Materials." EPA is the primary agency for Federal efforts to support State and local governments in response to an actual or potential discharge and/or release of hazardous materials following a major disaster or emergency. In such circumstances, there may be a presidential declaration of a "major disaster" under the Robert T. Stafford Disaster Relief and Emergency Assistance Act (the Stafford Act). The Stafford Act provides for Federal assistance to State and local governments when a major disaster overwhelms their ability to respond effectively to save lives; protect public health, safety, and property; and restore their communities.

Under the NRP, in the event of a terrorism attack EPA may receive a task assignment from DHS and, if a Stafford Act event occurs, a mission assignment may come from FEMA, now within the Department of Homeland Security. However, under the Stafford Act, mission assignments are designed to be primarily for an initial short period of time, normally no longer than sixty days, and may be with or without reimbursement. Under the NRP, even without a Stafford Act declaration, EPA could respond under its own authorities and funding. In the case of the attack on the World Trade Center, EPA's actions were conducted in accordance with mission assignments from FEMA.[3]

---

[2] PDD 62 reaffirmed Presidential Decision Directive 39 (PDD 39), which, among other things, specified that the "laws of the United States assign primary authority to the States to respond to the consequences of terrorism; the Federal Government provides assistance as required." Both PDD 39 and PDD 62 are classified documents. The quotations are from unclassified synopses prepared by the Department of Justice.

[3] EPA previously has corresponded with you on several occasions concerning the specifics of the response to the September 11 terrorist attack. The following letters are attached: February 22, 2002, letter from Administrator Christine Todd Whitman; April 25, 2002, letter from Regional Administrator Jane M. Kenny (referenced attachments not enclosed given their length); July 29, 2002, letter from Jane M. Kenny; and March 5, 2003, letter from Jane M. Kenny.

I hope this additional background information regarding the Agency's authorities and its appropriate role in the event of a terrorist attack is helpful to you. If you have further questions, please contact me or your staff may contact Carolyn Levine, in EPA's Office of Congressional and Intergovernmental Relations, at (202) 564-1859.

Sincerely,

Ann R. Klee
General Counsel

Enclosures

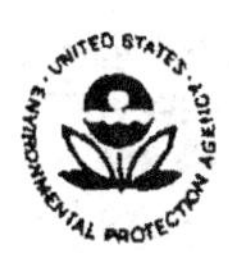

UNITED STATES ENVIRONMENTAL PROTECTION AGENCY
WASHINGTON, D.C. 20460

FEB 22 2002

The Honorable Jerrold Nadler
U.S. House of Representatives
Washington, DC 20515

THE ADMINISTRATOR

Dear Congressman Nadler:

Thank you for your letter of January 23, 2002, regarding environmental conditions in New York City following the September 11 terrorist attacks. I share your concern for the people of Lower Manhattan, and also believe that the federal government has an important role to play in both the monitoring of current conditions and in trying to develop reliable information about the health effects on people living and working in the areas surrounding the World Trade Center site.

The environmental and public health issues resulting from the attacks of September 11th have no precedent in the experience of this Agency or the federal government. Given the extraordinary challenges, I am proud of the work of our dedicated employees in response to the attack on our Nation. Our Agency's personnel were on the scene almost immediately, and have been working closely with the Federal Emergency Management Agency (FEMA) since President Bush's declaration of a federal disaster at the World Trade Center. The President's declaration triggered the Federal Response Plan and directed FEMA to coordinate various federal, state, and local agencies and the American Red Cross in carrying out thirteen distinct Emergency Support Functions. The Environmental Protection Agency (EPA) has served in a supporting role to the City of New York and the State of New York, consistent with the Federal Response Plan and mission assignments from FEMA.

In response to your concerns that authority was not properly delegated to the City of New York, it is important to note that under the Federal Response Plan local governments have primary responsibility for responding to an event. Those governments however, can turn to the federal government for assistance where they need it. In this event, the City of New York asked, through FEMA, that EPA assume lead responsibility for monitoring the outdoor conditions at and around the site of the event and for decontaminating the streets and other outdoor public areas. As explained in the enclosed Summary of Current Actions from October 6, the City assumed responsibility for indoor testing and the reoccupancy of buildings.

The EPA responded to the City's request promptly and thoroughly. Since September 11th, EPA personnel have established numerous monitoring stations around Lower Manhattan that have analyzed both air and particulates for various toxins known to cause long-term risks to public health. In addition, we have made every effort to disseminate to the public the results of our monitoring. Our Web site (www.epa.gov) contains the results of all of our outdoor monitoring dating back to September. We have endeavored to present the information gained from our monitoring in a form readily available and accessible to the general public.

2

Let me also address your concerns about the cleanup of federal buildings. EPA did not set a more stringent standard of cleanup for these federal buildings, and the lobby cleanup was consistent with the New York City Department of Health advisory. After noting significant amounts of dust tracked into 290 Broadway and 26 Federal Plaza by workers responding at the World Trade Center, the General Services Administration asked EPA to clean the lobbies. The work was done by EPA contractors using HEPA vacuums already operating in the area. As outlined in the enclosure, EPA collected seven air samples at 26 Federal Plaza and six air samples at 290 Broadway, and found results below levels of concern. No other specialized cleanup was conducted on the upper floors of either building.

In regard to your concern that EPA guided residents to the New York City Health Department for direction on cleanup of homes, this was appropriate since traditionally, the health agencies make recommendations to the public on health-related issues. Our Agency also advised residents in frequent public appearances, press releases, and phone conversations on our 24-hour hotline, that if they had more than minimal dust they should hire a certified asbestos cleanup contractor. For those with only minimal dust, EPA also continued to recommend wet wiping, mopping, and HEPA vacuuming in these situations, consistent with what the City's recommendations.

Despite the City's best efforts to address indoor environmental issues, many concerns and challenges remain. I am committed to providing additional assistance to the City and its residents and stand ready to do so. I will also be working with our local, state, and federal partners to establish a Task Force on Indoor Air in Lower Manhattan so that we can move quickly to address the remaining concerns we all share.

All this being said, I believe that Congress and the Administration need to revisit the issue of authority and responsibility for indoor environmental conditions in the wake of a terrorist attack. While the current practice is to vest responsibility in local and state governments for indoor environmental conditions, perhaps this approach is not appropriate in the wake of an event like September 11th. I would welcome the opportunity to work with you and your colleagues to explore this issue further. Until such determinations are made, however, we will continue to offer our full support to the City of New York and stand ready to assist with any further requests they may make for our assistance in dealing with indoor environmental issues.

Again, thank you for letter noting your concerns. I know that we share the same goal of protecting, as best we possibly can, the people of the United States from the environmental hazards that may exist following a terrorist attack. You have my pledge that we at EPA will continue to work as hard as we can to meet that obligation to the people of New York and be ready to meet it should the need arise in the future. Please contact Michele McKeever at 564-3688 with any further questions.

Sincerely yours,

Christine Todd Whitman

Enclosures

USEPA Air Analytical Results from 9/13/01 Sampling Event

26 Federal Plaza: Seven air samples were collected at the 26 Federal Plaza (13th, 26th,38th,39th floor and in the lobby). The asbestos concentrations ranged from non-detect to 0.0072 fibers/cc (south lobby). Data results are less than the OSHA Permissible Exposure Limit of 0.1 fibers/cc.

290 Broadway: Six air samples were collected at the 290 Broadway (8th, 22th, LL-1, LL-2 and Lobby). The asbestos concentrations ranged from non-detect to 0.0133 fibers/cc (LL-1).

One Chase Plaza: One outdoor air sample was collected at the one chase plaza; the asbestos concentration was 0.0098 fibers/cc.

Methodology
Air samples were analyzed by TEM EPA 40CFR763 AHERA .
Dust samples were analyzed by PLM - EPA-600 R-93/116.

attachments to 2/22 letter to Nadler from Whitman

Summary of Current Actions

ICS 201

06Oct01

Critical Issues

9/30/01:

Roof Debris: EPA spoke to COE on 9/30/01. COE has discussed issue with NYC and NYC is not asking for Federal assistance. The Federal Response Plan assigns responsibility to the COE under ESF-3, Public Works and Engineering, to provide Federal assistance for debris cleanup and removal.

Residential sampling/reoccupation: On 9/30/01, EPA spoke to US Public Health Service and NYSDOH who have been discussing issue with NYCDOH. NYC will not be requesting State or Federal assistance for residential sampling or reoccupation issues. The Federal Response Plan assigns responsibility to the U.S. Public Health Service under ESF-8, Health and Medical Services, when state and local resources request Federal assistance for medical and public health assistance.

Communications

10/03/01

Ground 0: Portable radios are now operational for communications between Mobile Incident Command Post (MICP) and Ground 0 field personnel. All other comms out of the MICP must still use phones, with installed lines being used primarily and cellular phones secondarily. Six installed lines will be installed into the new EPA/CG trailer...projected installation date is Monday, 8 Oct 01.

Landfill: A VHF repeater link has been installed to provide comms between the landfill and the EPA Command Post in Edison, NJ. Radios must be on Channel 1 in order to communicate between the two command posts. Local comms at the landfill will be on Channel 2.

Additional info.: Although the frequencies being used are dedicated to the USCG, they are NOT digitally encripted (secure), therefore no sensitive issues may be transmitted and professional terminology MUST be displayed.

GROUND "0" BRANCH

Wash Group 1

10/05/01:

Contractors are maintaining 18 operational wash stations. Contractors are monitoring and recording the number of personnel using their respective wash stations.

10/06/01:

Demob of station B1 currently in progress. Truck washing operations being transferred from Turner to Miller Environmental at request of NYC so that Turner will not be washing their own trucks. Group Supervisor responsibilities being transferred to Lt. Boyles from Lt. Brannan who demobs this date.

Personnel Assigned: CG: 15   Contractor: 70

Projected future actions: All vehicles must be out of parking lot at West and Vesey by 0500 hours, 10/07/01 due to paving operations to create pad for EPA Command Post.

Wash Group 2

10/06/01:
Status to be determined.

Personnel Assigned: EPA: 4   Contractor: 6

SuperVac Group:

10/05/01

Continued working west side of West Street near Millennium Park. Completed EPA parking lot. Will be working night shift only for the week-end beginning this evening. Received requests to vac city parks including Washington Market, Bowling Green, City Hall and Battery.

10/06/01

Completed vac and laser wash of D.O.T. lot and West St. south of Thames St. Night only operation continuing. Tonight Rector St. will be washed.

Personnel Assigned: EPA: 5   EarthTech: 36

Projected future actions: OSC Weden will be coordinating additional vac and wash sites with NYC DEP with EPA Operation Deputy. EPA in Edison will be coordinated mapping of vac sites.

Disposal Group

10/05/01:

Received no report.

10/06/01:

Received no report.

Personnel Assigned: EPA: 2   START: 9   EarthTech: 16

Projected future action: IAW hazwaste disposal plan, conduct above ground HAZMAT recovery; conduct underground storage tank reclamation; stage vac-trucks @ pier and landfill

ICS 201 Summary of Current Actions   Updated as of 1700, 10/06/01

Outfall Group

10/05/01:

Continued monitoring areas along likely trajectories. Nothing to report.

10/06/01:

Continued monitoring areas along likely trajectories. Nothing reported.

Personnel Assigned EPA: 6   EarthTech: 7

Projected future actions: Continue boat patrols for debris/evidence at outfalls. Identify precautionary measures to intercept materials prior from reaching outfalls.

SAMPLING BRANCH

Lower Manhattan Group

10/05/01:

Completed two rounds of real-time monitoring...all stations except for one due to demolition near buildings 4 and 5. Nothing significant to report. Changed asbestos pumps and picked up filters. Four tedlar bag samples taken. N. Norrell walked area with city officials assessing locations for portable weather stations. C. Jimenez collected 10 samples at landfill.

10/06/01:

No Bulk sampling conducted. Two sessions of real time monitoring conducted with no significant readings. Changed asbestos monitors. Collected 1 tedlar bag sample in smoke plume at Ground Zero. Installed 2 self sufficient satellite weather monitors (1 at Stuyvesant High School & 1 on roof of Century 21 building).

Personnel Assigned: EPA: 6   CG: 1   Contractor: 21

Projected future actions: Sampling as needed if requested by DEC or Port Authority. Bulk sampling will be conducted at landfill on 10/07/01. Bulk asbestos sampling will resume on building rooftops in and around the ground zero area either on the afternoon of 10/07/01 or the morning of 10/08/01.

ICS 201

Organic/Metallic Group

10/05/01:
No activity.

10/06/01:
No activity.

Personnel Assigned   EPA: 1   RST: 0

<u>**Projected future actions**</u>: Conduct sampling IAW sampling plan. Will continue to sample the landfill every other day.

Data Assessment Group

10/05/01: Continue distributing as outlined.

10/06/01: Continue distributing as outlined.

Personnel Assigned   EPA: 3   Contractor: 10

Projected future actions: Continue distribution of data and data summaries IAW plan.

Ambient Air Group

10/05/01:

ORD: 6 filter samples for particulates and successful download of real-time data at locations A, C, K, and 290 Broadway.

10/06/01:

ORD: Changed filters and downloaded continuous measurements at locations A, C, K and EPA building at 290 Broadway.

Personnel Assigned EPA:4   DEC: 6   Contractor: 1

<u>**Projected future actions**</u>: Conduct sampling IAW sampling plan in near zone and general population

LANDFILL BRANCH

Landfill Sampling Group

10/05/01:

Data Rams logging every 15 minutes and checked hourly. SKC pumps continuously running.

10/06/01:

Six Data Rams logging every 15 minutes and checked hourly. Thirteen SKC pumps continuously running.

Personnel Assigned   EPA: 1   CG: 5   REAC: 3

Projected future actions: Continue sampling IAW sampling plan. Start taking bulk samples for asbestos at landfill.

Landfill Wash Group

10/05/01:

Fine tuning wash stations; all staffing will be in place tomorrow.

10/06/01:

Personal hygiene station to be operational by 1700, vehicle washing station not operation at this time. Vehicle washing operation should begin on 10/07/01.

Personnel Assigned: EPA: 1   CG: 5   IT: 12

Landfill Disposal Group

10/05/01:

Received no report.

10/06/01:

No activity reported.

Personnel Assigned   EPA: 1

ICS 201 Summary of Current Actions   Updated as of 1700, 10/06/01

ICS 201 Summary of Current Actions   Updated as of 1700, 10/06/01

EPA Edison Command Post

Personnel Assigned   EPA: 25   CG: 15   Other: 8

Total Personnel Assigned

EPA: 65   CG: 41   Other: 234

Finance

Total ESF 10 ceiling:

12,000,000.00   Total Inter agency Agreement (IAG)

171,756.67   Coast Guard   (through 05 Oct)

Contractor Obligations:

3,000,000 (approx.)   Cleanharbors

3,000,000   Miller Environmental

1,500,000   I.T. Corporation

Total Spent to date: $7,671,756.67

Ceiling Remaining: $4,328,243.33

ICS 201

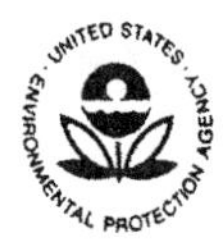

UNITED STATES ENVIRONMENTAL PROTECTION AGENCY
REGION 2
290 BROADWAY
NEW YORK, NY 10007-1866

APR 25 2002

Honorable Jerrold Nadler
U.S. House of Representatives
Washington, DC 20515

Dear Representative Nadler:

This is in response to your March 7, 2002, letter to Administrator Christine Todd Whitman concerning the Environmental Protection Agency's (EPA's) actions following the September 11 terrorist attacks on the World Trade Center (WTC) in New York City, which has been referred to me for reply.

I certainly understand your concerns and those of your constituents regarding indoor air quality in lower Manhattan. EPA is addressing those concerns through a multi-agency Task Force on Indoor Air. We are prepared to engage in constructive discussions about them with you and others.

I would now like to respond to the questions in your letter. In response to your first and third question, EPA was tasked by the Federal Emergency Management Agency (FEMA) under the Federal Response Plan (FRP) through mission assignments to perform duties as described below (your second question). These response actions were directed by six predesignated Region 2 On Scene Coordinators (OSCs). There names are in the attached list. While there were hundreds of other OSCs and non-OSCs from EPA throughout the country and the U. S. Coast Guard who assisted in the WTC response, these six OSCs were primarily responsible for directing activities. These OSCs reported to Bruce Sprague, Chief, Response and Prevention Branch, EPA's Emergency and Remedial Response Division.

To respond to your second question, EPA was tasked with four major mission assignments from FEMA, which are described in detail below and functioned as outlined in Emergency Support Function-10 (ESF-10) under the Federal Response Plan (FRP). In addition to its mission assignments, EPA had staff assigned to the Disaster Field Office of FEMA and the NYC Emergency Operations Center through late November. EPA was supported in its mission on this disaster by the U.S. Coast Guard National Strike Force and personnel from other EPA locations including the National Environmental Response Team. The following are the major mission assignments made by FEMA to EPA, in support of New York State and the City of New York, and a description of the tasks that were performed by EPA during the period from September 11 through December 31, 2001:

Mission Assignments 02 & 18 - Assess all hazardous substance and oil releases throughout the NY/NJ metropolitan area resulting from the WTC attack. Support to include, but not be limited to, providing personnel and equipment to conduct sampling, staging, securing and disposing of hazardous materials and oil releases; coordinating necessary response actions to limit the spread of contaminated materials; assisting in removal and disposal of contaminated materials; vacuuming and power washing; and providing air monitoring for response and cleanup operations and at disposal locations. Personal protective equipment was provided for federal, state, and local responders and volunteers. Under these mission assignments, assistance was also provided in checking for natural gas leaks and other explosive hazards in buildings used by financial firms to allow retrieval of necessary records for relocating business operations.

The scope of this mission assignment, as written, is clearly quite broad. However, FEMA, EPA, the city and the state of New York met on October 9, 2001 regarding the issue of assessment of potential contamination in indoor residential spaces in lower Manhattan. At that meeting, the city stated that it would not be requesting state or federal assistance for residential sampling or reoccupation issues. This sort of interagency coordination is expressly contemplated by the Federal Response Plan and the National Contingency Plan. See, *e.g.*, 40 CFR § 300.130 (h) and (i).

Mission Assignment 03/04 - Outfall activities, water runoff activities from area of Ground Zero. Under this assignment, EPA looked for possible evidence of releases of hazardous material or oil into the Hudson and East Rivers.

Mission Assignment 31/33 - Development and implementation of a physical hygiene plan (wash operation) for workers at Ground Zero and Fresh Kills Landfill.

Mission Assignment 34 - Construction of the Central Wash Station, West and Vesey Streets.

After December 31, 2001, EPA signed three Interagency Agreements (IAGs) with FEMA to continue performance of the following tasks:

Air monitoring at Ground Zero, Fresh Kills Landfill, New Jersey and the five boroughs of New York City.

Hazardous waste collection and disposal, vacuuming and power washing, if appropriate.

Workers and vehicle wash operations at Ground Zero and at Fresh Kills Landfill.

I have enclosed copies of the FEMA Mission Assignments and the IAGs referred to above.

With respect to your sixth and seventh questions, EPA used the nationally-accepted polarized light microscopy (PLM) method to analyze samples of the dust in lower Manhattan. The analysis was used to characterize the nature and extent of the outdoor asbestos contamination. The PLM analysis more than adequately indicated the widespread presence of asbestos in the dust. Based on this analysis, EPA took a blanket approach and removed all dust/debris regardless of whether sampling results indicated that the material contained asbestos. Additional TEM analysis would not have altered our response.

No bulk dust sampling was conducted by EPA at 290 Broadway. The sampling conducted on September 13 by EPA at 290 Broadway was limited airborne asbestos sampling, which was analyzed using the TEM methodology. For airborne asbestos sampling, we have used both transmission electron microscopy (TEM) and phase contrast microscopy (PCM) methods for analysis. EPA's landlord, the General Services Administration (GSA), took dust samples at 290 Broadway, which they analyzed using the TEM method.

In your January 23, 2002 letter, you asked for documents "detailing the justification of the cleanup of 290 Broadway and 26 Federal Plaza." As we previously explained, the lobbies of the two federal buildings were vacuumed to pick up dust tracked in by response workers. The vacuuming was done before EPA received the results of the dust samples taken by GSA, and no further cleaning was done after we received the data. The GSA results did not serve as a justification of the actions and were not even considered in responding to your initial request.

In response to your eighth question, I have attached a number of documents reflecting that EPA officials advised residents that they should hire a certified asbestos cleanup contractor. EPA's advice on this issue was reported in numerous press accounts. In addition, I attach a New York City Department of Environmental Protection Notice, which EPA used as the basis of its advice to residents at a series of public meetings and in response to telephone inquiries from the public.

Regarding your ninth question, the term "minimal dust" is a term of art, and we did not otherwise define it. We advised anyone who had more than a minimal amount of dust to employ professional asbestos contractors to clean their space. We believed that advice to have been both prudent and pragmatic.

Regarding your tenth question, we have made no statements about who ultimately should pay the costs of cleaning up indoor residential spaces in lower Manhattan.

In response to your eleventh and final question, EPA did not "delegate" its authorities or responsibilities with respect to the WTC collapse, nor did we at any time consider ourselves as having been "relieved" of any of our responsibilities.

As Administrator Whitman stated in her February 22, 2002 letter to you, EPA is committed to providing additional assistance to the city and its residents and stands ready to do so. EPA is collaborating with our federal, state and city partners to address ongoing concerns about indoor air quality through a multi-agency task force. The group has already made

5

considerable progress. With EPA's guidance, the New York City Department of Environmental Protection will remove residual debris from rooftops and building facades in lower Manhattan. EPA will conduct field work to assess cleanup techniques and provide information to guide ongoing cleanups. All of the involved agencies are working together to assess the cleaning that has been conducted and to develop testing criteria.

Lastly, I believe you are mistaken in your understanding of the terms of the Temporary Restraining Order (TRO) issued by Judge Roberts in *Martin v. Whitman*, alluded to in the final paragraph of your letter. The TRO, which has since been lifted, has no bearing whatsoever on our decision not to participate in the hearings held by Mr. Martin, and our decision certainly did not represent a violation of that order.

Sincerely,

Jane M. Kenny
Regional Administrator

Enclosures

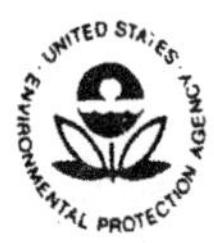

UNITED STATES ENVIRONMENTAL PROTECTION AGENCY
REGION 2
290 BROADWAY
NEW YORK, NY 10007-1866

JUL 29 2002

The Honorable Jerrold Nadler
U.S. House of Representatives
Washington, DC 20515

Dear Representative Nadler:

I am writing to update you on the progress the U.S. Environmental Protection Agency (EPA) has made since my letter to you of April 25 concerning post-9/11 environmental issues in lower Manhattan. I also want to respond to questions that you and others have raised about the extent to which EPA's indoor air response activities will be consistent with the National Oil and Hazardous Substance Pollution Contingency Plan, 40 C.F.R. Part 300 (the NCP). I know these issues are vitally important to you, as they are to me.

EPA continues to work supporting federal, state, and New York City efforts to recover from the federally declared disaster resulting from the September 11 attack on the World Trade Center. We do this under the authority of the Robert T. Stafford Disaster Relief and Emergency Assistance Act (Stafford Act) and in accordance with the applicable procedures and policies of the NCP. Our current focus is to address indoor air concerns through an indoor dust cleanup and air sampling program for residential spaces in lower Manhattan. I want to reassure you that EPA will implement a comprehensive program to ensure that lower Manhattan residents are protected from potential exposures to harmful dust and debris residuals. EPA will run this program in cooperation with the Federal Emergency Management Agency (FEMA), New York State, and New York City. We will use all the tools available, including appropriate aspects of the NCP, to achieve this goal as expeditiously as possible.

EPA is in the process of implementing three programs related to indoor air in lower Manhattan residences. These programs will be funded by FEMA under the Stafford Act, specifically Sections 403 (Essential Assistance) and 407 (Debris Removal).

<u>Components of the Indoor Air Residential Assistance Program</u>

First, EPA is directing a Confirmation Cleaning Building Study by collecting samples in a building that had only minimal cleaning since the attack, employing and evaluating various cleaning techniques. This project is under way, and field work should be completed in the next several weeks. Second, EPA is directing a Background Study to provide monitoring data on

2

indoor air contaminants in residences nortl of 2 j Street, which were not affected by the collapse of the WTC, so that such data may be compared with data obtained in residences in lower Manhattan. The contractor is in place for this study, and access has been granted for some of the sampling locations. Third, EPA, along with the New York City Department of Environmental Protection (NYCDEP), is providing for the monitoring and cleaning of lower Manhattan residences through the Indoor Air Residential Assistance Program - World Trade Center (WTC) Dust Cleanup. Pursuant to interagency agreements under the Stafford Act, FEMA is providing or will provide funds to the city, which used its emergency contracting authority to enter into contracts for a hotline contractor to register residents for the indoor dust cleaning program, and will be contracting with certified asbestos cleanup contractors to professionally clean apartments, as well as with Project Monitors to oversee the cleaning contractors. The actual cleaning and monitoring will be carried out by NYCDEP contractors, under the direction and oversight of EPA, in coordination with the city. FEMA and EPA are in the process of entering into an interagency agreement to support EPA's activities in this program.

We will evaluate the information and data that we gather in the Confirmation Study and the Background Study, as well as the results of a peer review of a draft technical document on World Trade Center Contaminants of Potential Concern, as the cleaning and monitoring activities proceed. We will use these data to determine whether any program adjustments or modifications are needed. As we have discussed, this approach of conducting studies and cleanups in parallel is necessary because of the scientific complexities of dealing with indoor environments and the need for timely response to the potential threat to public health and welfare. We have limited indoor sampling protocols, health benchmarks, background data for urban areas (especially Manhattan), correlations of dust to air exposures, etc. We are using cleanup methods effective for asbestos and fibrous materials and expect that these will be effective for any other particulate matter that may pose health concerns. We will do sampling for airborne asbestos in every residence we are asked to clean or test, but we will also do sampling for metals and dioxin in a subset of spaces. This will give us information on additional substances of potential concern. If the study work we are doing indicates that we need to modify our cleanup approach, we will do so. But at this time we feel it is appropriate to begin to clean residential spaces.

As you are aware, under the Indoor Air Residential Assistance Program -WTC Dust Cleanup, lower Manhattan residents will be given the option of requesting either cleaning followed by sampling, or sampling alone. To date, more than 3,500 residents have requested one or the other option.

<u>Relationship of the Indoor Air Residential Assistance Program to the National Contingency Plan</u>

You have asked whether the Indoor Air Residential Assistance Program - WTC Dust Cleanup will be conducted in a manner consistent with the NCP. As I noted in my April 25 letter, the NCP applies and is in effect whe. ̇ th̄ Federal Response Plan – the document providing the structure for a coordinated response under the Stafford Act – and some or all of its Emergency Support Functions (ESFs) are activated. [See 40 C.F.R. § 300.3 (d).] As also noted in my letter, ESF-10 (the Hazardous Material Annex) of the Federal Response Plan is applicable to this disaster response. ESF-10 states, "The NCP serves as the basis for planning and utilization of federal resources..." ESF-10 anticipates the potential for unique situations, in that it contemplates response "...to actual or threatened releases of hazardous materials not typically responded to under the NCP but that, as a result of the disaster or emergency, pose a threat to public health or welfare or to the environment." [See ESF-10, section I.B.4.] In such situations, "[a]pplicable policies and procedures in the NCP will be adhered to..." (emphasis added). [See ESF-10, section IV.B.1.f.] In this instance state and local government entities have asked EPA to provide technical lead and oversight of actions to address potential indoor air/dust cleanups for residential dwellings. This activity is consistent with Stafford Act Sections 403 and 407 and is coordinated by FEMA's Federal Coordinating Officer.

In developing the Indoor Air Residential Assistance Program - WTC Dust Cleanup, EPA has relied on the existing data, the intergovernmental collaboration process, and discussions with scientific, technical, and medical professionals and concerned community members. We believe this is appropriate given the urgency and scope of the actions needed to help restore lower Manhattan to pre-9/11 conditions.

The Indoor Air Residential Assistance Program -WTC Dust Cleanup responds to a disaster involving a release that is most certainly not typical, not only because of the terrorist act that led to the release but also because of the unique challenges posed by the presence and potential presence of WTC dust in thousands of lower Manhattan apartments. When the WTC collapse occurred, there was a release of asbestos, a hazardous substance, to the environment. The debris and pulverized dust from the collapse affected many structures in lower Manhattan to varying degrees. This release was documented by bulk dust sampling done by EPA; approximately 35% of bulk dust outdoors contained greater than 1% asbestos, which is a regulatory definition of asbestos-containing material (ACM) under federal, state and local statutes. The ACM was deposited in a very variable manner, that is, samples of bulk dust/debris, taken virtually adjacent to each other, had differing levels of asbestos. We believe that the dust materials that reached the interiors of structures was likewise variable in its deposition. In addition, some of the material may have contained asbestos at levels of concern for long-term risk, even though it may not have exceeded 1% ACM. Given that there are over 20,000 residential units in lower Manhattan, specifically identifying which of them were affected by amounts of dust potentially causing long-term health effects would be time- and resource-intensive. In addition, as I stated earlier, making risk exposure assessments in indoor environments is very complex. The variability of the WTC debris/dust material and the manner in which it affected building interiors adds another layer of complication.

4

In deciding upon a cleanup program for lower Manhattan residences we considered the following:

- the complexity of sampling dust material for quantities of hazardous substances and the lack of scientific consensus on how to do so;

- the absence of standards that have broad scientific support which correlate airborne exposure routes to dust containing hazardous substances; and

- the absence of health- or risk-based standards for dust.

In addition, we had to consider how we could gauge the residual impacts of cleanups already undertaken by residents who returned to their homes. All of the above have substantial uncertainty or controversy surrounding them.

Federal, state, and city health and medical professionals supported a program that addressed the need for cleanup assurances without the time, expense, and uncertainties associated with a location-specific sampling and risk assessment approach. EPA also consulted with environmental health and science experts in the academic and research sector on this basic approach. Though there were many questions and a desire for more data collection, they generally acknowledged that a broad-based cleanup program was an appropriate response.

For these reasons, and in consultation with FEMA, New York City, and New York State, EPA has determined that rather than taking a risk-based approach to each residential unit or building, we will instead clean any lower Manhattan apartment based on residents' request.

The NCP, pursuant to CERCLA, authorizes EPA to undertake or direct cleanups in response to releases or threatened releases of hazardous substances into the environment. [See Attachment, Note 1.] As background, you should be aware that sections of the NCP, for example, those dealing with long-term response, are simply not applicable here – for instance, 40 C.F.R. Sections 300.430 and 300.435, addressing remedial investigations and feasibility studies, selection of remedy, remedial design and remedial action, operation and maintenance, and attainment of 10^{-4} to 10^{-6} cancer risk levels. [See Attachment, Note 2.]

Consistent with the atypical aspects of the release and the response work that we face in lower Manhattan, to the extent practicable and appropriate we are proceeding with this program in a manner consistent with the NCP. Let me give several examples.

- Our efforts are consistent with the NCP provisions regarding the respective roles of different federal agencies and organizational elements, such as the National and Regional Response Teams and the On-Scene Coordinator. [See 40 C.F.R. Part 300 Subpart B.]

We are responding to residents' concerns in a manner consistent with the NCP. [See, for example, Section 300.415(n) of the NCP, 40 C.F.R. § 300.415(n) ("Community relations in removal actions").] In brief:

> (a) we have designated spokespersons for our programs related to the attack on the WTC, who respond to inquiries and keep the community informed regarding our actions. They will make available data related to indoor air concerns in lower Manhattan, providing such data in a manner that does not divulge the address of a given residence or the name of a given resident;

> (b) we have been meeting and will continue to meet with public interest groups or other interested or affected parties, as appropriate, to solicit their concerns and information needs, and find out how or when citizens would like to be involved in the process;

> (c) we are preparing a communications strategy which will address many of the concerns raised in the meetings with community members and other relevant information and will specify the community relations activities that we expect to undertake during the Indoor Air Residential Assistance Program -WTC Indoor Dust Cleanup; and

> (d) we have established at least one local information repository in lower Manhattan (290 Broadway) which is accessible to the public. At that location we will make available documents which have formed the basis for our actions.

Working with the city we have made changes to the scope of work which will form the basis of the city's contractor solicitation for the cleanup and testing program based on concerns raised by interested members of the public.

We have developed the clearance level (that is, the risk-based clean up goal) to determine when cleaning can cease at a residence under the Indoor Air Residential Assistance Program -WTC Dust Cleanup. The development of this level has been consistent with the NCP. For example, under the NCP, removals performed either by EPA with Superfund monies or by responsible parties need to attain applicable or relevant and appropriate requirements (ARARs) "to the extent practicable considering the exigencies of the situation." [Section 300.415(j) of the NCP, 40 C.F.R. § 300.415(j).] For the Indoor Air Residential Assistance Program -WTC Dust Cleanup, it was determined that there were no directly applicable standards. So, as is a common practice in removal actions under the NCP, we have developed a risk-based clearance number for asbestos in air, taking into consideration other standards. We have consulted with peers in the scientific community to assure that this level represents an extremely protective long-term risk guideline.

The attack on and collapse of the World Trade Center was a truly unprecedented event, far different from every other federally declared disaster. As such, it warrants a unique response that is consistent with federal disaster plan guidelines but also adopts a bias toward immediate action to protect the health and safety of the residents of lower Manhattan. I believe very strongly – as does the Administrator – that we must act swiftly to address the real and immediate concerns of residents while adhering to the applicable and appropriate provisions of the NCP. The goals of the NCP - protecting the public from environmental releases of dangerous substances – will be fully served through the decisive and comprehensive approach we are taking.

As I close, I want to assure you that the EPA personnel involved in the World Trade Center Indoor Dust Cleanup Program have significant experience in overseeing contractors and cleanups, making judgments about risk, and properly communicating about such matters with the public. We are taking this program very seriously and are devoting a huge amount of our staff resources to ensuring that it is carried out in a safe, protective, and responsive manner.

If you have any questions regarding this matter, please contact me at (212) 637-5000, or Kathy Callahan, Assistant Regional Administrator for NYC Response and Recovery Operations, at (212) 637- 3116.

Sincerely,

Jane M. Kenny
Regional Administrator

Enclosure

Notes

1. As I noted in my April 25 letter, while the NCP authorizes EPA to take actions to address the release and threatened release of a hazardous substance into the environment, Section 300.400(i)(3) of the NCP states, "Activities by the federal and state governments in implementing this subpart are discretionary governmental functions. This subpart does not create in any private party a right to federal response or enforcement action. This subpart does not create any duty of the federal government to take any response action at any particular time."

2. Many have commented that this risk range, used for remedial sites under CERCLA, is the one that should apply to the Indoor Air Residential Assistance Program - World Trade Center Dust Cleanup Program. As discussed elsewhere in this letter, EPA has developed a particularly stringent clearance level for asbestos in lower Manhattan residences. Nonetheless, for the following reasons, even if this were a remedial site, the 10^{-6} cancer risk -- which is a "point of departure" referenced in the NCP -- would not be used because it is impracticable to achieve. All protocols chosen for the Indoor Air Residential Assistance Program - World Trade Center Dust Cleanup Program are designed to reach the lowest level of detection that is reasonable with established methods. For asbestos, the sampling and analytical protocols chosen are designed to attain risk estimates of 1×10^{-4}. To reach estimates of 1×10^{-6}, extraordinary modifications would have to be employed to either significantly increase the volume of air being sampled or to go to extraordinary expense to analyze many more grids on each sample filter. An increase in the sample volume, through an increase in flow rates from 10 to 15 liters/minute to 500 to 1,000 liters/minute would lower the detection level. However, the only equipment available to operate at these rates are large units that are impractical to bring into a residence. Achieving flow rates this high has not been tested using the sampling protocols, and there would be a high likelihood of compromising the sampling filters. To achieve detection levels consistent with 1×10^{-6} risk values by running the equipment for longer periods of time would require increasing the period of sampling from 8 hours to 33 days. These two issues make it impractical to achieve a 1×10^{-6} detection level.

UNITED STATES ENVIRONMENTAL PROTECTION AGENCY
REGION 2
290 BROADWAY
NEW YORK, NY 10007-1866

MAR - 5 2003

The Honorable Jerrold Nadler
U.S. House of Representatives
Washington, DC 20515

Dear Congressman Nadler:

I am writing in response to your letter concerning the Environmental Protection Agency's (EPA) Indoor Air Residential Assistance Program that the EPA is jointly conducting with the City of New York's Department of Environmental Protection (DEP), using disaster funding provided by the Federal Emergency Management Agency (FEMA). In particular, you sought information about the legal and scientific bases for aspects of the program.

I am pleased to report that our cleaning and testing program is going well. As you know from prior correspondence from me, our goal is to protect lower Manhattan residents from potential exposures to residual dust that may contain pollutants from the collapse of the World Trade Center (WTC), and to provide residents with information that will help them feel comfortable in their homes. EPA has received approximately 5045 requests for cleaning and testing of apartments and an additional 1,219 requests for testing only. As you note in your letter, we have begun work in both areas. To date, over 1,568 apartments have been cleaned and tested, and 450 have been tested. Testing of 1589 residences addressed either by testing alone or cleaning and testing have revealed results below the EPA clearance level (see Note 1, Enclosure 1). Seventeen residences had samples that exceeded the clearance level, and an additional 70 percent had results that could not be determined because of filter overload or other testing-related problems (see Note 2, Enclosure 1).

One area about which you request information concerns personal protective equipment (PPE) for cleanup workers. I note that all work performed under the program is being done in compliance with applicable laws and regulations, including but not limited to regulations issued by EPA, the United States Department of Labor Occupational Safety and Health Administration (OSHA), the New York State Department of Labor (NYSDOL), and DEP. The contract entered into by DEP for cleaning requires that only a NYSDOL-licensed asbestos contractor and only DEP and NYSDOL-certified workers would be allowed to perform any of the cleaning activities under this contract. This requirement also applies to any subcontractors involved in the cleaning. The contract entered into by DEP for the project monitors (who are responsible for, among other things, overseeing the cleaning work and insuring that work is satisfactorily completed) requires the use of experienced personnel certified by New York State. I also note that we have worked with OSHA to assure that contractors meet OSHA regulatory requirements. For instance, pursuant to our discussions with OSHA, we have implemented personal air monitoring for a specified number of the cleaning employees (see Note 3, Enclosure 1).

Under the contracts for the program, residences and common areas (including elevator shafts) of residential buildings that appear to have been minimally impacted by dust and debris from the collapse of the WTC are addressed using different procedures than those required in the event visual inspection indicates the presence of significant accumulations of WTC dust and debris. In the former instance, procedures referred to in the contracts as "Scope of Work A" apply; in areas of significant accumulation "Scope of Work B" is utilized. Under Scope of Work B, PPE is utilized. As you point out, the use of PPE by cleanup and monitoring workers is not required under Scope of Work A.

There were reasons for this. On June 14, 2002, Patricia K. Clark, the Regional Administrator of OSHA Region 2, issued a Negative Exposure Assessment (NEA), consistent with their regulations, based on sampling in the immediate vicinity of the WTC (Enclosure 2). Regional Administrator Clark indicated that her assessment included both the workers directly involved in WTC debris removal and those exposed to heavy settled dust accumulations in buildings immediately bordering Ground Zero.

On August 5, 2002, Christopher Ward, the DEP Commissioner, wrote to Regional Administrator Kenny about whether DEP and NYSDOL requirements apply to Scope A work (Enclosure 3). In his letter, Commissioner Ward said that Scope of Work A situations are not "asbestos projects" or "minor asbestos projects" under DEP's Asbestos Rules, and further, with regard to Article 30 of the New York State Labor Law, which DEP enforces in New York City, such cleanings are not "abatement projects." By its letter, DEP confirmed that it would not require PPE in the Scope A scenario (see Note 4, Enclosure 1). Of course, should the personal air monitoring of workers indicate risks to the workers, we would immediately consult with OSHA and revisit this decision.

You also request information concerning the focus of the program solely on residential spaces. I note that EPA has been providing information and advice regarding commercial and educational spaces in lower Manhattan. For instance, we have facilitated an understanding of cleaning and testing in the public schools. The cleanup program in the New York City public schools has been implemented by the New York City Department of Education, which has taken primary responsibility for testing and cleaning the schools. FEMA is providing financial support for this effort. Some parents of students expressed great concern about the appropriateness of the cleanup being done. As part of our ongoing efforts, EPA agreed to organize and facilitate a meeting with appropriate agencies and interested and involved parents regarding details of the Department of Education's cleanup program. EPA also has reviewed the sampling results obtained through private contracting by the Department of Education for Stuyvesant High School. EPA's review found that the air sampling results at all locations in the school meet the clearance criteria set forth in the Asbestos Hazard Emergency Response Act (AHERA) for re-entry into schools following an asbestos abatement project.

As I indicated to you in my July 29, 2002 letter, the authorities under which the program is operated and funded clearly state that the response actions undertaken/to be undertaken are discretionary functions. While the owners and occupants of commercial spaces have been able to rely on commercial insurance resources and on other governmental programs, tenants and residence owners have not had the same degree of resources available to address testing and cleanup (see Note 5, Enclosure 1). EPA remains confident that the cleaning procedures recommended to the public for residential and commercial spaces following the collapse of the World Trade Center are effective. Our view has been confirmed by data from the program. While the recommended cleanup methods may, in some cases, have to be applied more than once, they are effective. We are continuing to evaluate the monitoring results and how they may apply to cleanup efforts previously undertaken in non-residential buildings. We will keep you informed of our progress.

There remains much to be accomplished; however, I believe that with the cooperation and assistance of all our partners and with input from the public, we will achieve our goal of protecting the public from potential exposure to residual dust that may contain pollutants and providing them with information that will help them feel comfortable in their homes.

I look forward to working with you, as well as other members of the community, as we address the indoor air concerns of the residents of lower Manhattan. If you have any concerns please contact me at (212) 637-5000 or have your staff contact Peter Brandt at (212) 637-3657.

Sincerely yours,

Jane M. Kenny
Regional Administrator

Enclosures

Enclosure 1
Notes

Note 1:   As referenced in prior correspondence with you, we have developed the clearance level (that is, the risk-based cleanup goal) to determine when cleaning is effective in a residence participating in the Program. For the Program, there are not any directly applicable standards that have broad scientific support which correlate airborne exposure to dust containing hazardous substances. Accordingly, as is common practice in removal actions under the National Oil and Hazardous Substances Contingency Plan, we have developed a risk-based clearance number for asbestos in air, taking into consideration other standards. We have consulted with peers in the scientific community to confirm that the chosen clearance level is a protective long-term risk guideline.

Note 2:   Initial personal air monitoring was performed by the Cleaning Contractors, in accordance with OSHA requirements, at a minimum of one employee per shift per residence per quadrant for the first 10 weeks of cleaning operations. Currently samples are being taken at one sample per quadrant per day. Results of this sampling are being provided to both the EPA and OSHA and are also available to the employees or their designated representative in accordance with 29 CFR 1910.1020 and 29 CFR 1926.1101.

Note 3:   In a residence not meeting the clearance level where only testing was conducted, EPA recommends that the home be cleaned and re-tested. In a residence where both cleaning and testing were done, EPA attempts to identify potential sources of pollutants and then re-clean and re-test the home to meet the clearance level.

Note 4:   I am informed that under New York State law, the use of PPE in asbestos projects is addressed in the New York State Labor Law and its implementing regulations, and in the Rules of the City of New York. PPE is required only for workers involved in "asbestos projects" or "minor asbestos projects" under DEP's Asbestos Rules, and involved in "asbestos projects" under the New York State Labor Law.

Note 5:   For instance, governmental financial assistance, including but not limited to grants and low interest loans for commercial property owners, was and still is available through the Small Business Administration, New York State Economic Development, New York City Economic Development Corporation, and FEMA. For further information on governmental funding for commercial and business properties, you may contact Joseph Picciano, Acting Regional Director, FEMA Region 2 at (212) 680-3609.

U.S. Department of Labor

Occupational Safety and Health Administration
201 Varick Street
New York, New York 10014
Tel. (212) 337-2378
Fax:(212) 337-2371
OSHA Website Address: http://www.osha.gov

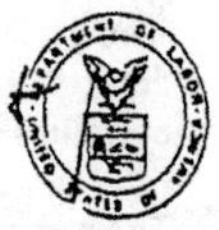

June 14, 2002

Kathleen C. Callahan
U.S. Environmental Protection Agency
Deputy Regional Administrator
290 Broadway
New York, NY

Dear Ms. Callahan:

This is in response to your latest electronic request addressed to David J. Ippolito, in which you sought a written description of OSHA's asbestos monitoring data for the assessment and selection of personal protective equipment for use by contractors who will be included in your residential clean-up program.

29 CFR 1926.1101 presumes worker exposure to asbestos in the construction workplace for specific work operations until this presumption is rebutted by air monitoring or until the employer has obtained a Negative Exposure Assessment as defined in this standard. As you know, OSHA activities at the WTC site have included assisting the New York City Department of Design and Construction and the New York City Fire Department (co-incident commanders) in characterizing exposures to many contaminants, including asbestos.

Results from that sampling activity indicate that worker exposures to airborne asbestos have been, and continue to be, very low relative to the applicable limits. As of June 10, OSHA has taken 1,398 airborne asbestos samples (both personal and area) on and around the WTC site. Those samples were analyzed by Phase Contrast Microscopy (PCM) for total fiber counts, which counts all fibers as defined in the OSHA standard, not just asbestos fibers. Of the 1,398 samples taken, only 157 revealed exposure in excess of OSHA's applicable Permissible Exposure Limit (PEL) of 0.1 fiber per cubic centimeter. However, when discriminating counting techniques and/or Transmission Electron Microscopy (TEM) analysis was performed on these samples, the asbestos fiber count was always less than half of OSHA's PEL.

In addition, OSHA's Manhattan Area Office has initiated an enforcement local emphasis program (LEP) to monitor cleanup activities in damaged buildings surrounding the WTC site, which we believe represent the heaviest of the settled dust accumulations. The boundaries of this LEP are: Chambers to the North, Broadway to the East, Rector to the South and Hudson River to the West. The air and bulk samples collected during those monitoring inspections contain no detectable levels of asbestos. In summary, as of June 11, 2002, twenty-five bulk samples of settled dust and debris taken from six of these surrounding buildings as part of this LEP/building debris removal all were found to be non-detected for asbestos. Twenty-five air samples, the majority being personal samples, taken in these same buildings to assess exposure on workers who performed various construction tasks and building cleanup operations were found to be non-detected for asbestos. For more specific information of the results of this sampling and the buildings sampled please see the attached addendum.

The sum of these sample results constitutes a large pool of historical data representing employee exposure to airborne asbestos dust and constitutes a **Negative Exposure Assessment** as defined by Section 29 CFR 1926.1101, paragraph (a). That assessment includes both the workers directly involved in the debris removal at the WTC site, as well as those exposed to heavy settled dust accumulations in buildings immediately bordering ground zero. Therefore, while the settled dust originating from the WTC collapse may contain asbestos exceeding 1 percent, the dust poses a very low risk to the workers who disturb it.

Once a negative exposure assessment for asbestos has been obtained pursuant to 29 CFR 1926.1101, then workers would not be required to use any protective clothing or respiratory protection. Therefore, based on this historical asbestos sampling data obtained at Ground Zero and the surrounding affected buildings, OSHA's assessment for the EPA cleanup of residential apartments would not require workers to use any respiratory protection or protective clothing.

OSHA does not discourage the voluntary use of respiratory protection or other personal protective equipment that is provided to employees in the interest of worker safety and health. However, please remember that OSHA's respiratory protection standard 29 CFR 1910.134 requires that employers may provide respirators at the request of employees or permit employees to use their own respirators if the employer determines that such respirator will not in itself create a hazard. If the employer determines that any voluntary respirator use is permissible, the employer shall provide the respirator users with the information contained in 29 CFR 1910.134 Appendix D. Please also remember that 29 CFR 1910.134 (e) *medical evaluation* and (f) *fit-testing*, require that employees be medically evaluated and fit tested before using any respirator other than a "dust mask" (filtering face piece). Employees who voluntarily use only a "dust mask" or filtering face piece would not be required to be medically evaluated or fit-tested. Employers who voluntarily provide protective clothing for their workers should also be aware that protective clothing worn at elevated temperatures may create additional hazards such as heat stress / heat stroke. Workers using such clothing may need frequent breaks and plenty of fluids.

Should you require any additional information or need further clarifications, please feel free to contact me at (212) 337 - 2378.

Patricia K. Clark

Regional Administrator
Region II

ADDENDUM - A - MANHATTAN OSHA AREA OFFICE
LEP ASBESTOS SITE SPECIFIC INSPECTION DATA

90 West Street:Activity:
Samples taken:
4 bulks for asbestos: All were ND for asbestos
2 bulks taken on 2nd fl ground & 2nd fl stairway debris
2 bulks taken from overhead Thermal System Insulation

3 personal air for asbestos: All were ND for asbestos
Total Fibers range from ND - .1800 f/cc

Activity: Electricians working in the basement

102 North end Avenue:

Samples taken:
3 asbestos (air) were taken: All were ND for asbestos
Total fibers range from 0.0230-0.0620 f/cc

Activity: 3rd phase of cleaning area - cleaning hotel rooms using HEPA vac

3 World Financial Center:

Samples taken:
6 bulks for asbestos were taken: All were ND for asbestos
(4) 4th fl -NW side of building (WTC debris)
(2) 6th fl - Area already cleaned -took samples as precaution

3 personal air samples for asbestos: All were ND for asbestos
Total fibers range from .0960 - .270 f/cc

Activity: 2 samples employees bagging office material in area contaminated from WTC collapse
1 sample employee cleaning HVAC system

1 World Financial Center:

Samples Taken:
5 bulks for asbestos were taken: All were ND for asbestos
4 personal air samples for asbestos: All were ND for asbestos

Activity: Carpet mastic removal

130 Liberty Street:

Sample Taken:
6 personal air samples conducted for asbestos   All ND for asbestos
2 Area samples taken in the plaza area   All ND for asbestos

Activity: Carpenters performing renovation
                                     operation/clean up

130 Cedar Street:

Samples Taken:
4 personal air samples conducted for asbestos   All ND for asbestos
10 bulk samples taken on floors 2 through 11 for asbestos   All ND for asbestos

Activity: Asbestos abatement contractor removing debris
                                     subject to Governor's emergency order

Department of
Environmental
Protection

59-17 Junction Boulevard
Flushing, New York
11373-5108

Christopher O. Ward
Commissioner

August 5, 2002

Hon. Jane Kenny
Regional Administrator
U.S. Environmental Protection Agency, Region II
290 Broadway, 17th Floor
New York, NY 10007

Re: World Trade Center Indoor Dust Cleaning
    Program

Dear Ms. Kenny:

I am writing to advise you that DEP's Bureau of Environmental Compliance (BEC) has reviewed the draft "Cleaning Contract Scope of Work" for the World Trade Center Indoor Dust Cleaning Program (Draft - 8/2/02) (copy attached).

With regard to "Scope of Work A", which sets forth the procedures to be employed where minimal dust accumulations are present, BEC has determined that such cleaning work does not constitute an "asbestos project" or "minor asbestos project" as those terms are defined in the DEP Asbestos Rules, Title 15, Chapter 1, Rules of the City of New York §1-02.

Further, insofar as DEP is authorized pursuant to §24-146.2 of the New York City Administrative Code to enforce Article 30 of the New York State Labor Law and the regulations adopted thereunder, BEC has determined that cleaning work undertaken pursuant to "Scope of Work A" does not constitute an "asbestos project" as defined in §901 of the New York State Labor Law and 12 NYCRR Part 56-1.4(o).

Sincerely,

Christopher O. Ward

Thomas G. Day
Senior Vice President
Government Relations

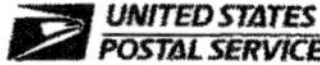

UNITED STATES
POSTAL SERVICE

September 21, 2005

Mr. Robert Briggs
Clerk
Subcommittee on National Security,
  Emerging Threats and International Relations
Committee on Government Reform
House of Representatives
Washington, DC 20515-0001

Dear Mr. Briggs:

This is in response to the questions for the record from the April 5 hearing, "Assessing Anthrax Detection Methods."

The first question pertains to the priority schedule for the Biohazard Detection System (BDS) installation at U.S. Postal Service facilities nationwide. The Postal Service began nationwide installation of the BDS in April 2004. As of September, 1,131 systems have been installed in 226 facilities. All units required to cover letter mail (1,361 units at 282 sites) will be installed by the end of November. With the exception of a few sites that require extensive site preparation work, the Ventilation and Filtration Systems equipment also will be installed by the end of March 2006.

The second question pertains to the scheduled dates of BDS installation at the V Street facility in Washington, D.C. On May 20, BDS installation was completed at the 3055 V Street facility, which is the warehouse. On May 27, BDS installation was completed at 3300 V Street, the Annex.

Thank you for your continued interest in postal matters. If we can be of any more assistance, please don't hesitate to let us know.

Sincerely,

Thomas G. Day

475 L'Enfant Plaza SW RM 10226
Washington DC 20260-3500
202-268-2506 Fax: 202-268-2503
www.usps.com

9780160750847